"This is a marvelous book, so real and realistic, around the issues of food and solutions in how to meet what we eat with care and mindfulness. Annie Mahon has offered us not only recipes for eating but recipes for living. I am so grateful."

—Roshi Joan Halifax, Abbot, Upaya Zen Center

"Beautifully written and compulsively readable, this book is a feast of compassion for the struggling, weak, suffering sides of us. It's heaped full of comfort and practical help for anyone who struggles with painful emotions, self-doubt, and the desperate urge to not feel what we are feeling. Highly recommended, with a deep bow."

—Ann Weiser Cornell, *The Radical Acceptance of Everything* and *Presence*

"With courage and humility, Mahon reminds us that food—rather than being fraught with disconnection and discontent—can help us come to our senses. As we cook and eat, she gently encourages us to listen to our bodies, to reclaim our original natures, and to recall our deep and intimate membership in the wider world."

—Tovar Cerulli, *The Mindful Carnivore*

"Annie's compassionate writing addresses an issue of struggle for so many—every day eating. Through the sharing of her journey and struggles, you'll gain insight into your own relationship with food, discover ways to work with disordered eating, and learn practical tips to adjust your palate and habits for overall well-being."

—Kimberly Wilson, *Tranquility du Jour Anthology* and *Tranquilista*

"Take one raw, hilarious, searingly honest, and compulsively readable memoir; fold in a wise, compassionate guide to mindful eating; and blend it with a delicious vegetarian cookbook. That's the recipe for Annie Mahon's nutritious new book *Things I Did When I Was Hangry*. Whether you devour it in one sitting or savor it for days in small bites, this book is a feast for the spirit."

—Anne Cushman, *Moving into Meditation*

Things I Did When I Was Hangry

Things I Did When I Was Hangry

*Navigating a Peaceful
Relationship with Food*

Annie Mahon

PARALLAX
PRESS

Berkeley, California

To my mom and dad without whom my world would not exist. And to all of the women and men who suffer because of their relationship with food.

Parallax Press
P.O. Box 7355
Berkeley, California 94707

Parallax Press is the publishing division of the Unified Buddhist Church, Inc.
© 2015 by Annie Mahon

Cover and text design by Nancy Austin Design, Oakland
Cover image © LHF Graphics/Shutterstock.com
Author photo © Max Hirshfeld

Library of Congress Cataloging-in-Publication Data is available upon request.

ISBN: 978-1-937006-98-3

1 2 3 4 5 / 19 18 17 16 15

Contents

Introduction

I WROTE THIS BOOK BECAUSE I didn't really know how or what to eat until I began practicing mindfulness. Once I did, I became aware of how many others experience suffering around eating as well. I hope this story, of one family's experience, will help. It has been more challenging for me to be joyfully present in my kitchen than in any other room of my house. My goal for the last two decades has been to relearn how to nourish myself with food. Mindfulness has been my best teacher.

Eating is not a winning game, but if it were, I would never win the award for "Most Mindful Eater." I might, however, win for "Most Improved," or maybe "Valuable Team Player." I have overcome a pattern of eating disorders and held the hand of several friends and relatives as they walked various paths to healing their own eating disorders. Along the way, my relationship with food and cooking changed.

The basic practice of mindful cooking and eating is this: In each moment, if your mind wanders away from what you're doing, pause, breathe, and return your attention to your physical experience, whether it's preparing food or eating it. It's really that simple.

I had dinner a year ago with a woman who is considered an expert on mindful eating. In the weeks leading up to our meal, I worried about her seeing that I wasn't a real "mindful eater." Fortunately, my companion didn't seem to notice when I overloaded my fork or talked with my mouth full. We simply enjoyed our conversation and our food. I realized that this was an example of how I had wasted years of my life worrying about what and how I would eat, judging myself and expecting others to judge me too. This habit has kept me from enjoying my food and my life more times than I can count. Mindfulness has not dissolved this habit, but it has made me more aware of it, and now this worrying happens much less often.

The aim of practicing mindful cooking and eating is to increase the joy of cooking and eating. When I mentioned to a friend that I was writing this book, she assumed that I cook every meal at home joyfully and eat every meal with my family in mindful bliss. She thought I might judge her way of cooking and eating because it wasn't like that. Wrong. It isn't the end of the world if my family orders in pizza, has pancakes for dinner, or talks nonstop through a meal. It's okay if we don't agree about food and what to eat. There isn't a right way to do it, and it doesn't help anyone to be judged for how and where they eat.

These days, I rarely obsess about what to cook and eat. I eat mostly intuitively and enjoy taking care of myself and my loved ones by creating and eating healthy meals that taste good. I still work on remembering to cook with awareness and to eat sitting down without distractions. There's a saying that resentment is like drinking poison and hoping the other person will die. My relationship with food has been like this: I was angry at food for its power over me, and so I ate it without enjoying it. Of course, the one who suffered was me.

When I was a young child, I was much more in touch with my food. I remember enjoying the look and smell of green peas as they rolled around my plate, their texture when I squished them with the back of my fork, and how it seemed to take forever to finish the one spoonful I had been served.

But, like many of us, my upbringing, my genes, and the cultural pressures of the times conspired to change my relationship with preparing and eating food. By the time I reached puberty, I was already unable to enjoy eating because of my preoccupation with my weight. Preparing food wasn't as interesting either; I had other, seemingly more important, things to do. I no longer listened to what my body wanted and needed to eat.

As I got older, life got busier and I had even less time for cooking and eating. I began to eat out more often or to buy food that was processed or prepared. I was lost more often in my mind rather than experiencing life through my senses in the present moment. To begin the process of transformation, I had to be able to stop running around, stop distracting myself, stop thinking so much about food, and start experiencing food the way I had as a child.

I have been very lucky to have had enough food to eat throughout my life, while many people in this world have not. The idea of bingeing, purging, or purposeful starving would be incomprehensible to some people living in the world now, and certainly to a lot of our less well-off ancestors. As I reflect on the difficulties that my family and I have experienced around food, I am also reminded over and over again of how extremely fortunate we have been to have each other and to have all the resources that we need to survive.

Lastly, in addition to my mindfulness meditation and yoga practices, I have had the benefit of a good therapist through the years who has specifically helped me around eating disorders. I'm not sure I would have been able to make the changes I have without the time I spent with her.

After years of practice and therapy, I am still not one hundred percent mindful in the kitchen. Sometimes I eat lunch in front of my email, while reading the newspaper, or even while driving to teach a meditation class. Sometimes I make my lunch and it's eaten before I even realize it. What my mindfulness practice does is keep me from freaking out or beating myself up. More often than not, I simply laugh at myself and try again next time. And that feels like progress to me.

There are many positive side effects to mindful cooking and eating, but this book is not about how to lose weight, look younger, or become a top chef. It's about learning how to show up for the moments of your life, and it is likely that you spend many of them in the kitchen or around food. My hope is that, in sharing my story, practices, and recipes, you will find help restoring your own natural capacity for nourishment with food and be able to reduce suffering both in yourself and in the world.

About the Recipes

THE RECIPES IN THIS BOOK were shared with me or were born from other recipes that I modified or tweaked to make them more to my liking. Some were first made for me by someone from whom I learned something about mindful eating, like my grandma or my friend Yo.

Some recipes were accidentally modified because I didn't have the necessary ingredients, didn't want to use the suggested ingredients, or wanted to simplify the recipe for my family, and they ended up tasting great. The dishes in this book are all relatively easy to make (except maybe the dumplings) and are excellent for practicing your mindful cooking even when you don't have much time. They are all vegetarian, but not all are vegan. Some originated from recipes in the newspaper or books that I read once and later re-created from memory. Like the children's game Telephone, those recipes are slightly different every time I make them.

I hope that you'll make the recipes your own in the same way; there is very little that can go wrong other than not liking the taste. If that happens during your explorations, so what? Kitchen mess-ups just offer us another chance to practice our mindfulness. Get curious about recipes the way you might have played with your chemistry set or with the colors in a finger painting.

If you don't have one ingredient, try a similar one in its place. If you like more fire, add some cayenne pepper or other fresh hot peppers, or toss in a little spicy salsa. And always feel free to incorporate what's in season and looks good at the farmers' market or grocery store that week. As long as it's edible, you can't hurt anyone by playing with your ingredients.

There are no hard and fast rules. As you will see in the following chapters, your rules will derive from your contemplation of the world and how you want to live in it. The more you look inward, the more you will learn, and the clearer you will be about how you want to cook and eat. And as you cook more often with awareness rather than distraction, you will be able to learn how food works, and gain confidence in yourself and your mindful kitchen.

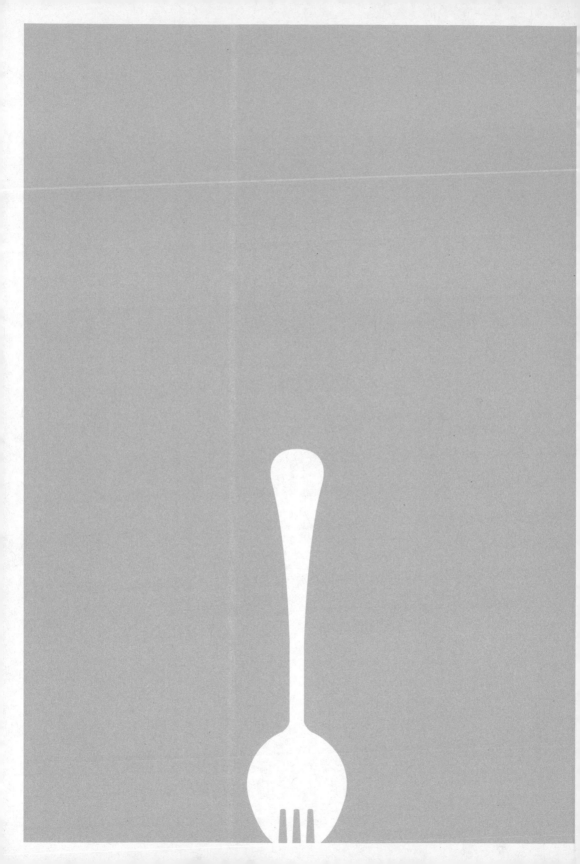

1.

STARTING
from SCRATCH

Ring the bells that still can ring. Forget your perfect offering.
There is a crack in everything. That's how the light gets in.

—LEONARD COHEN

It's 1977 and I am a high school junior. I am buying munchies (a.k.a. binge food) at the local A&P supermarket. As usual, the checkout aisle is lined with magazines and mini-books like *Your Sun Signs* or *Fifty Styles for Problem Hair* packed into racks with *Betty & Veronica* comics. Though I know better than to buy any of the junk sold in the checkout aisle, that day I instinctively and impulsively pick up a tiny book and scan its pages while I wait in line. In the two minutes before the cashier with the Farrah Fawcett haircut greets me with her predictable "Hey there," this book has whispered something vital into my discontented heart. I sense that I need whatever it's dispensing. This book might just save my life.

THE BOOK I BOUGHT (or possibly shoplifted) that day was called *Self-Hypnosis* by Leslie M. Lecron. It was the size of my palm. I was drawn to it because I had been the subject of hypnosis at a free event, and had subsequently allowed myself to be hypnotized in the back office by the owner of the Bob's Big Boy restaurant where I waitressed. This could have ended badly, but fortunately was rather banal. Still, I was intrigued by the feeling of deep relaxation I'd had when I was hypnotized, a feeling at that time I could only compare to having smoked a big bowl of weed.

Hypnosis, self-hypnosis, and, later, meditation allowed me to loosen my grip on all the things I was trying so hard to control—my appetite, my weight, my acne, my place in my family and with my friends. I never felt that I fit in anywhere. When I was practicing self-hypnosis, my troubles didn't seem so big and menacing. I could simply breathe in and out, my body and mind slowly relaxing. When I guided myself into self-hypnosis, I was a more content version of me.

Each day I sat cross-legged on the burnt orange carpet in my bedroom following the instructions in the little book. Relaxing my body and slowing down my breathing... I am getting sleepier and sleepier... Every time I did it, I felt great. No one in my family and certainly none of my friends—most raised in strict Catholic families—would have understood this, and I never told anyone about this strange habit. After some time, I decided self-hypnosis required more effort than just popping a pill or smoking a joint. So when I left for college in 1979, I didn't take my budding meditation practice or even my little book with me. But I never completely forgot that feeling of peacefulness, which slept like a seed inside me, waiting to be watered.

I Love Food

I grew up in Sterling Heights, a blue-collar suburb of Detroit, given the nickname "Sterile Whites" because of its lack of diversity. My favorite food was macaroni and cheese, which I liked to eat with green peas. As a youngster I was really in touch with my food. I loved the peas' bright green color, slightly earthy smell, and mushiness; the macaroni took effort to chew, and the peas popped open in my mouth, their vegetableness infused with the sweet flavor of melting butter, like waves washing over my tongue.

Creating food was equally thrilling. Mixing the cheese sauce into the cooked macaroni or squeezing thick ketchup onto steak was a blast. Spreading peanut butter on bread to make a peanut butter and jelly sandwich was messy, and eating it was fun. I would rip it into pieces, lick the edges that dripped off the crust, or open the whole thing up and eat it from the inside out. Even spooning baby food into my little sister's mouth was exciting and playfully messy. I not only loved the food itself, I also loved its sensuality.

In those early years, I related to food entirely through my senses. I ate with my body, not just my mind. I was really there with my food, not lost thinking about it—or obsessing over it. Much later, that relationship turned upside down and was the root of decades-long dysfunctional eating habits.

Crazy-Making

When I was about ten years old, I began to change. I was a quiet, bookish, sensitive child (and pretty much still am), who liked to make people happy.

And I remember the first time I let social conditioning control my actions rather than living from my intuition: when I lied in order to please someone else. I went to school wearing a new and quite adorable orange wool dress that stopped mid-thigh, a stylish mini-dress, in fact. On the playground at recess, another girl told me that my dress was pretty. I was proud of that dress, and was about to agree, but an unfamiliar voice in my head chimed in and reminded me that if I accepted a compliment, it would elevate my own status at the expense of the other girls. It said, "You wouldn't want that, would you?" It suddenly seemed wrong to look good. So I looked down and muttered, "Oh, this ugly dress isn't as nice as yours…" I insulted myself in order to protect her and gain her approval, a seed that took root and spread to all areas of my life as I grew up. Pretty soon I barely knew what I really thought and felt. I just knew that compared to other people, I wasn't very good, competent, pretty, or smart.

My mom and dad did the best they could under the circumstances. Their own childhoods had been filled with alcoholism, illness, and death. My dad lost both of his parents, refugees from the Armenian genocide, by the time he was fifteen. My mom's father was seriously ill most of her childhood. Both of my parents taught at a large community college; my mom taught writing, and spent countless evening and weekend hours grading papers, volunteering with nonprofits, and fundraising for local politicians. My dad taught economics, ran a small newspaper, and was on the Macomb County Board of Commissioners.

I was the third of four children. I had an older sister, Maggie, and an older brother, Patrick. When I was six, my younger sister Julia, a bubbly brown-eyed cherub, was born, which made me sometimes an adoring older sister and other times a jealous little brat.

Our dinner table was often the source of drama. My parents had polar opposite relationships to food. My dad was always trying to keep himself from eating something. My mom, a strict vegetarian, was a pillar of control. She fed her husband and us four kids copious quantities of food that she didn't or wouldn't eat. To manage his weight, my dad tried lots of fad products and pills, including liquid protein until it killed a couple of people and was banned. So while my mom ate her nightly baked potato with steamed broccoli and low-fat cottage cheese, we chowed down on steak, chicken and dumplings, macaroni and cheese, bagels, and boiled veggies.

My dad tried hard not to finish everything on the table, but he generally cleaned his plate, the serving dishes, and whatever his kids hadn't gobbled down before he looked over. He didn't want to eat all that, and his suffering sometimes caused him to lash out at us. He was angry with my mom for cooking so much food, my sister for using the wrong fork (and stressing him out), me for leaving food he *had* to eat, and my brother for leaning back in his chair. I dreaded coming to dinner.

My mom had her own method of coping with the chaos. She believed that if you talked about something, it became more real. So if you didn't talk about troubling things, they would go away. Unpleasant emotions like sadness, fear, and anger were best managed by rewriting the story that produced them or by simply denying their existence.

When I begged my parents to stop fighting, my mom would say, "We're not fighting, we're just discussing." When my brother punched or choked me, she told herself (and me) that we were only "playing." Mom only saw the positive, allowing her to believe that everything was fine even when it wasn't. Later I discovered a way to use my mom's practice of "looking for the good" to help me generate more happiness, as long as I didn't also ignore or dismiss my suffering.

What I learned from all of this was how to ignore the very real sensations and feelings I was experiencing in the present moment and live only in my thoughts and stories about them. By focusing more and more of my attention on food, I could avoid feeling my unwanted emotions.

Social conditioning was another big factor in my food obsession. Then, as now, we were relentlessly bombarded with messages telling us to buy and eat—the wheels of our economic system can turn only when we remain at least a bit dissatisfied with ourselves. Late-night ads for Red Lobster restaurants, Little Caesars Pizza, and other food giants promote unhealthy supersized meals. According to a National Institutes of Health study, just seeing a food advertisement increases our likelihood to eat more snacks.[1]

In between those ads, we watch endless shows and movies that tell us just the opposite: that we can only be happy if we are ridiculously skinny. Women (and men to a lesser degree) are rarely depicted in the media or popular culture as having average body sizes and shapes.

Social media has further reduced our ability to accept our natural imperfections. We feel we have to compete with the seemingly flawless lives of our "friends" as advertised on Facebook timelines and in Instagram photos. Our discomfort with our bodies is epitomized by the slew of shows about losing weight (think *The Biggest Loser* or *Thintervention*) that shame "contestants" dealing with compulsive and binge eating disorders. I remember the one time I watched *The Biggest Loser*. A frightened contestant was wearing a large white tank top displaying her current weight in huge letters while the female trainer screamed, "I'm bored with your pathetic story... All I care about is that your ass gets smaller, that's all I care about!"

We've all consumed these paradoxical messages. We are supposed to eat for entertainment, comfort, or distraction from loneliness. But when we gain weight from all that food, we are shunned. No wonder so many of us forget how to eat in a mindful, natural way.

I wanted to fit in. So I tried to figure out how I should eat in order to be thin. Clearly food was the enemy, and I had to find a way to battle it in order to stay healthy and thin. I snuck into my parents' room every morning after they left for work to pilfer my dad's diet pills and laxatives from his underwear drawer. I tried the cabbage diet, the carrot diet, and the fasting diet. Like my mom, I eventually became a vegetarian, though I found many other ways to lose weight before that. In the process, I stopped enjoying food altogether. I was either "hangry"—tense and cranky from suppressing my natural hunger—or despairing when I gave in and ate "bad" food.

By the time I reached puberty, the only relationship I had with food was a resentful one. I was sure I was the fattest person in the room at five foot five and one hundred twenty pounds and I thought about my body size constantly. It was as if I were torn between my parents' two ways of eating—wanting to binge, like my dad, to escape from my angst, but also wanting to enjoy the kind of power my mom had over eating. Being thin got me attention from my dad and the boys at school, and I watched my little sister, only slightly larger than I was, denigrated because of her weight.

I restricted my eating whenever I could. Starting in junior high, I used my lunch money for drugs. I was given one dollar and twenty-five cents for lunch, and each morning I arrived at the school smoking area for a cigarette and to buy a one dollar hit of acid, mescaline, THC pills, or a joint. The remaining twenty-five cents bought me a roll and an ice cream sandwich. Eating food made me gain weight. Taking drugs gave me a momentary escape from a mind filled with insecurity, guilt, social awkwardness, and sadness. The choice was pretty easy.

Soon I learned that I could get a similar feeling of numbness from binge eating as well. Upset? Eat six bagels toasted with cream cheese. Worried about a boyfriend? How about a couple of cans of tuna mixed with gobs of mayo, some toasted pita-bread cheese sandwiches, and a frozen Sara Lee cake? I'd toast a bagel while stuffing tuna in my mouth, and while eating the bagel, start cutting the cake. I didn't really see, smell, or taste anything. I was in a binge trance.

I don't remember when I first learned how to purge after eating, but it seemed like the perfect way to have my cake and get rid of it too. I could eat as much as I wanted (like my dad) and still have control over my weight (like my mom). Starting in high school, this became my go-to way to manage strong emotions. I made sure there was a bathroom near every binge. At the end of a nasty binge-purge session, I was exhausted enough to finally rest. I felt a kind of temporary quiet not so different from the calm of self-hypnosis.

Food became my enemy and I became more and more isolated from my family and my friends. My bingeing and purging was a secret that I couldn't tell anyone. I even tried to keep it a secret from myself by shutting down my sensations as much as possible.

Watching TV and reading magazines like *Seventeen* and *Cosmopolitan* made me think that if only I were as thin as those women, everyone would love me and I would be forever happy and at peace. The inner critical voice was so loud that I couldn't hear very much else. The only way I knew to avoid feeling fat and unworthy was to stop eating and feel some control, or binge eat and feel nothing.

On the Outside

My family was different from the families of the kids I went to school with. Both of my parents had graduate degrees, while none of my friends' parents had gone to college. Most of my friends' mothers stayed at home, but my mom worked full-time. We lived in a 150-year-old farmhouse on three acres, and my friends all lived in brand new matching houses in a subdivision within shouting distance of each other. I knew I didn't fit in.

A lot of girls at school worried about their weight, but they seemed much saner than I was about it, and they all seemed thinner than I was. I felt alone with my hatred and anger toward food. To cope, I shut down my senses. When I wasn't bingeing, I was often mindlessly snacking. I ate while reading a book, doing a crossword puzzle, talking on the phone, and even while walking from one place to another. A bag of SweeTarts could evaporate during a chapter of *Little Women* or an episode of *The Partridge Family* without me noticing a single bite.

In high school I was tasked with making dinner on the nights my mom had a late class. I had one meal in my repertoire: broiled steak, microwaved baked potatoes, and frozen peas and it felt like a chore to prepare it. I had a love-hate relationship with food: I resented and tried to avoid it, even as it was my constant companion.

I didn't trust that I could control myself around food. In the sorority house when I was at the University of Michigan, the communal kitchen was locked every night. More than once I found myself leading a small band of women to break into the kitchen after a long night of partying. Each refrigerator was individually locked too, so we had to use long-handled spatulas to reach some of the booty. We polished off whatever we could grab—huge vats of egg salad, pasta, dinner rolls. In the mornings after such a binge, I felt physically sick and overflowing with guilt and shame. I felt so powerless over food, so I forced myself to atone for eating it by purging or restricting. Then I would be starving and hangry again and forced to binge. The cycle seemed endless.

One day early in my sophomore year, I had a craving bigger than any I ever had before. It was my first semester in the sorority. I told my roommate that I was desperate for egg rolls and she agreed to help me find some. This was before the Internet, so we consulted the Yellow Pages and had a dozen egg rolls delivered to the house. After devouring them without pause, I felt satiated for a minute. But something was still off. I went to see a doctor, accompanied by Jack, my boyfriend at the time. The doctor told us that I was pregnant. In that moment, I remember how I quietly closed and then locked the inner door of my thoughts and feelings. I didn't allow myself to feel anything except, "No, this can not happen to me." I felt determined, but otherwise I was completely numb. I told no one else.

I have always written about my life. When I was in elementary school, I traded pages of letters with friends at school. My longest "note" was fifty pages written to my friend Molly. In high school I started journaling, and wrote about the ups and downs of teenage life and love. On one page I would be ecstatic, the next self-loathing. When I found out I was pregnant, I wrote about it in my *Dear Ziggy* journal. And when we decided to have it terminated, I wrote about that too. There was literally no one in the world other than Ziggy that I felt safe telling. I thought my family would shame and punish me, and my sorority sisters would denounce me. I kept my secret inside.

To my horror, my sister Julia, only twelve at the time, discovered my journal during Christmas break and confronted me with her worries about my well-being. I denied everything, telling her I made it up. I tore out the relevant pages and burned them, convincing myself that it never happened and repressing the memory for more than a decade.

After this, my bingeing and purging only increased. Jack and I broke up, leaving me even more isolated. I was failing courses and abusing cocaine, weed, and alcohol regularly. It was a low point for me.

I had always felt pulled to the West Coast because it seemed more open and progressive than Michigan, so I decided to spend the following summer in the Los Angeles area living with my mom's twin brother, a brilliant but depressed nuclear physicist. I hoped I could find my tribe in California and finally feel like I fit in, so I arrived at my uncle Robert's house ready for a fresh start. When I knocked on the door, he opened it with his eyebrows drawn together and a snarl on his face. "I thought you were coming tomorrow," he said.

That beginning was a sign that California was not going to be the panacea I'd hoped. Robert lived twenty-five miles from the ocean on a cul-de-sac in the middle of residential suburbia with manicured lawns. This California was more uptight than any place I had lived before.

I also seemed to be the only person in the state without a car. During my first week I managed to figure out how to get to the shopping mall by bus and applied for jobs at most of the retail stores there without much success. My uncle was uncommunicative—I'd had no idea how depressed he really was until I lived there. One day I decided to bake some of my grandma's homemade bread as a way to connect with my senses and my family, and to bond with my uncle. He arrived home from work that evening ready for his usual solo meal, deliberately ignored my offer of fresh-baked bread, ate his dinner, and went to bed. I ate the bread alone. Confused and lonely, I punished myself for reaching out by vowing to eat only enough to survive for the rest of my visit.

I kept my promise to myself and lost more than twenty pounds over the next three weeks. I finally did get a job at the May Company store at the mall in the dress department, but I wasn't able to keep it because I had no transportation and extremely low energy.

I wasn't thin enough to be hospitalized, but I wasn't well. I spent all of my free time in my room watching TV and reading magazines, with a special focus on anything that would support my anorexic behavior. The first TV movie on the subject of anorexia, *The Best Little Girl in the World*, aired that summer, and I was riveted to the screen. Between the movie and all the subsequent media coverage, I learned new ways to control my eating, which in turn suppressed my feelings. After only four weeks, I decided I needed to go back to Michigan because I wasn't in my right mind. Without some human contact there was no telling how far I might take this punishment.

In the fall I took my food restricting back to school along with my other addictions. At a crowded Iggy Pop concert in October, someone passed me a joint. After taking a puff, I collapsed. I hadn't eaten in three days. My friends told me later that they carried me out of the concert unconscious. This wasn't the first time I had fainted from not eating, but it didn't stop me from starving myself.

The wisdom that had been so obvious to me as a young girl—that food was fuel for the body, a treat for the senses, fun to prepare, able to feed us in countless ways—was no longer accessible to me. As my eating disorder took over more of my life, I became further distanced from a mindful relationship with food. It was clear that even with all my weight changes, purging, and drug abuse, my parents either weren't aware or didn't know what to do about it. I knew I had to find a way to heal from my addictions to food—both bingeing and restricting—and alcohol and drugs, or I wasn't going to survive.

Macaroni and Cheese and Peas (*vegetarian and vegan options*)

This recipe grew from watching my mom make a cheese sauce hundreds of times. I never recorded it exactly, but it looks and tastes a lot like hers, especially if you use white wheat elbow pasta and orange sharp cheddar cheese.

INGREDIENTS:

½ pound, approximately 2 to 3 cups, of elbow pasta or any other smallish, hollow pasta, white or whole wheat

Cheese Sauce (see below)

paprika to taste

breadcrumbs (optional)

1 cup frozen peas

CHEESE SAUCE (NON-VEGAN):

1 tablespoon butter or margarine

1 tablespoon flour

¾ cup milk or heavy cream

4 to 5 ounces grated cheese. I prefer to use organic sharp cheddar, but you can use anything that has some sharpness to it.

salt, nutmeg, and/or paprika to taste

"CHEESE" SAUCE (VEGAN):

1 tablespoon Earth Balance or other vegan margarine

1 tablespoon flour

¾ cup soy, almond, or rice milk, unsweetened

4 to 5 ounces shredded Daiya soy cheese or other vegan cheese

salt, nutmeg, and/or paprika to taste

METHOD:

Cook the elbow macaroni according to package directions.

Preheat the oven to 350 degrees.

Make sauce as follows:

Melt butter/margarine in a medium saucepan.

Lower heat and add flour slowly, stirring with a fork until blended.

Slowly add milk or nondairy alternative and heat until almost, but not quite, boiling, stirring regularly.

Add most, but not all, cheese, one handful at a time, stirring constantly until sauce is thick and creamy.

Add spices to taste.

Mix sauce with the cooked pasta and pour into a casserole dish.

Cover with extra cheese. If desired, sprinkle breadcrumbs on top.

Bake for 20 to 30 minutes, or until bubbly hot and lightly browned.

Boil the frozen peas according to instructions on the package, and allow to drain.

Serve pasta with peas.

Serves 4.

Mom's Apple Crisp *(vegan)*

This is the dessert that my mom made most often at home—she gave me the recipe when I moved out of our house and I continue to make it for my family. It's easy and delicious. Mom made it with white sugar and "oleo" (ordinary margarine), but I suggest turbine sugar or maple syrup and soy margarine instead. The amount of topping ingredients can vary greatly depending on how much topping you like on your crisp.

INGREDIENTS:

4 to 5 apples: Granny Smith, or others with some tartness

1 to 1½ cups unbleached white flour or ½ cup flour and 1 cup rolled oats

1½ to 2 cups turbinado sugar or ¾ to 1 cup maple syrup

⅔ cup vegan margarine

¼ to ½ teaspoon cinnamon

¾ to 1 teaspoon salt

METHOD:

Peel the apples if you prefer skinless applesauce.

Core and slice the apples into medium-sized wedges.

Place apples into 9 x 12 baking dish until ⅔ full.

Sprinkle 1 to 2 tablespoons water and cinnamon over apples.

Mix together flour, or flour and oat mixture, and salt.

Add sugar (or syrup). Note that if you use maple syrup, the consistency of the topping may be mushy, but it will dry out in the oven.

Crumble topping onto apples.

Chop the margarine into flakes and add over the topping.

Bake 40 to 50 minutes or until liquid is bubbling and top is lightly browned.

Serves 9 to 12.

2.

COMFORT FOOD

The seed of suffering in you may be strong, but don't wait until you have no more suffering before allowing yourself to be happy.

—THICH NHAT HANH

I'm on a visit home from college for the weekend and on the way to the Lakeside Mall one Sunday morning with my sister Julia and my ex-boyfriend Jeff. We drive by a small Christian church. It looks really cute, so I tell Jeff to pull over and I make them both join me for the service. After a rousing sermon, the minister invites anyone who wants to "take Jesus into your heart" to come on down to the altar. I feel like I need someone or something to help me with my eating and addiction issues, so I impulsively get up and walk down the aisle with the other handful of people looking to get saved that day. People sing and clap while each of us has our head quickly dunked into the baptismal font. I walk back to my seat feeling hopeful but not much else. The transformation I had imagined didn't really happen.

BEING "SAVED" WAS EXCITING but ultimately didn't make my obsessions and addictions go away or change my eating behaviors. I liked the idea of church, and I went occasionally while in college, especially after a long night of binge eating or drinking. But I felt like a fraud when I sang hymns that said things like "Faith of our fathers, holy faith! We will be true to thee till death." I didn't know or care who these fathers were, and I certainly didn't feel connected to them. I just wanted some peace.

For as long as I can remember, I have had the clear belief that every one of us is equally part of God and that Jesus wasn't unique in having that quality. But I always remained anonymous at church so that I wouldn't have to explain or justify my beliefs to anyone. Years later, when I found mindfulness, I would learn how engaging with others in my spiritual practice was a crucial step in my willingness to be vulnerable and authentic. At this point, though, I was simply looking for a way to create space and calm in my mind, and going to church was the best I could do. I didn't make the connection at the time, but when I sat in a silent church I felt the same sense of calm that I'd had when doing self-hypnosis on the floor of my room.

My life took a sharp turn the first semester of my junior year. After the summer with my uncle in California, my mental state got worse. In addition to starving, bingeing, and purging, I found refuge with a fraternity boy who liked cocaine as much as I did. We were what they now call "friends with benefits." In addition to drinking heavily and smoking weed, we snorted cocaine as often as we could afford it, and then we fondled each other until we passed out.

Around that same time, my dad took me to his teacher's credit union to apply for a two thousand dollar student loan to help pay my college expenses. When the check arrived at my college address in November, the temptation was just too great for me. I cashed it and spent most of the money on cocaine. The remainder I used to buy some nice Christmas gifts for my family.

When I got home for the holidays that year, my parents asked for the loan money that they had been counting on to defray my college costs. I told them that I spent it all on Christmas gifts, which was clearly a lie. My parents interrogated me at our kitchen table, but I refused to confess; I was completely cut off from any feelings about what happened, and I just kept repeating my story. I was a terrible liar, and I suspect they didn't really want to know, because after that week they never mentioned it again.

At the sorority house that January, I moved in with Lynda, a sweet and funny young woman who was majoring in computer science. She was petite and quite thin, which I admired, and she was highly organized. I loved to watch her draw her computer science projects with colorful markers and gather stacks of computer cards together with a rubber band. It was 1982, and this was the full extent of my knowledge of technology.

One cold night during the first week of classes, my parents called me. They had just received a notice from the university that not only was I a second-term junior without a major, I had also been put on academic probation because of my failing grades. The school told my parents that if I didn't declare a major and improve my grades, I'd be expelled. As I listened to my mom's angry voice, I looked desperately around the room and saw Lynda on the floor diagramming a computer project. Impulsively, I interrupted my mom mid-sentence to tell yet another lie, "Well, actually, I have a major. It's computer science."

I hadn't taken a single class in this field and had no interest in it, but I knew that this would meet with their approval. At that moment, I would have done absolutely anything to avoid having to move home and deal directly with my eating disorder and addictions. Living in a state of constantly being hangry clearly wasn't helping me make wise decisions about my life.

In the sorority, eating disorders were accepted, and even admired. There were one or two severely anorexic women in our house, and we spoke about them with a mixture of revulsion and awe. I heard other girls throwing up in the bathrooms many times a day. Alcohol abuse was rampant, and while drug abuse was much less common, I was still protected by the sorority-girl image and I knew that no one there would ever confront me about my addictions.

The day after my parents' call, I visited my academic advisor, declared my major, and started taking speed so I could keep up with the workload. I was determined to stay in school. With the help of the drugs, I studied well into each night and managed to get through the next semester with the best grade-point average of my college career. Despite spending the rest of my time in college living on croutons with ketchup, Bloody Marys, and Scotch, I managed to graduate at the end of my senior year with a degree.

During my last undergraduate semester, I applied for and didn't get several computer-related jobs, and I once again panicked. Still bingeing, purging, and obsessing about what, when, where, and how to eat, I feared having to move back home. Just weeks before graduation, I applied for conditional admission as a graduate student in the computer science department at the university. I was accepted and given a grant for full tuition, with the condition that I would need to maintain a B-minus grade-point average for the next two years. I had very little interest in studying any more computer science, but was relieved to know I had somewhere other than home to be for the next two years.

With the stress of a graduate program I wasn't suited for, I began to smoke cigarettes and hook up with men I didn't care about. I stopped going to church, although I still liked to read about yoga and meditation when I came across a book or article. I thought about dropping out of school, but I couldn't envision what I would do instead. I mostly wrote and read poetry—Denise Levertov, Sylvia Path—when I needed spiritual support.

It was an unexpected friendship that helped me begin to really transform my relationship to my body and food. I met my friend Yo when I moved into an apartment on Fifth Avenue in Ann Arbor. He was a runner, bicycle racer, and he came from a Chinese family that loved to cook and eat. One beautiful fall day, he took me running, and when we reached the top of a long hill, I felt better than I had in years. I found that I got the same high from running that I did from smoking, so I quit smoking immediately.

Yo cooked real food in a real oven for me, and we talked about the tastes, smells, and history of the food we ate together. He reminded me of what I already knew, that food could be something to enjoy and savor rather than endlessly battle. Our relationship inspired me to begin to care about food again.

Although I continued to binge and obsess, Yo's influence helped me see that there could be another way to think about food. In that same rental house, I met a young man named Michael, who lived downstairs who also had an interest in cooking. We started dating and eventually rented an apartment together, and we prepared meals that not only tasted good, but looked beautiful as well. His mother was an exquisite homemaker who had instilled in him an awareness of the value of aesthetics in the home and at the table.

These two men helped me begin the process of relearning how to slow down and be with food in a sensual way. With them, food could be enjoyed in reasonable amounts and savored with friends. When Yo cooked homemade Chinese dumplings and we ate them together, I experienced the pleasure of accepting and savoring a generous offering from the cook. I had forgotten how to enjoy a meal mindfully, and these moments became touchstones for what was possible in my life. Though I hadn't yet stopped bingeing on and restricting food, I began to trust myself around food more often. Yo was one of the first people I was close to who didn't obsess about food, weight, or eating. Being around him allowed me to begin to question my own obsessions.

The more relaxed I became around food and in general, the less often I needed to binge. I didn't feel that Yo and Michael judged me as harshly as I had been judged by the other people in my life, including myself. As the months went by, I started to accept and like myself more. Between my new running habit and my increased self-acceptance, vomiting didn't seem as necessary as it had been before. Each purge made me feel ashamed and physically sick. By the end of that year, I had stopped throwing up entirely.

The Geographic Cure

Michael was a foodie before foodies were trendy. He liked good food, and together we explored the variety of restaurants in Ann Arbor. One of our favorite places was Zingerman's, then a brand new local spot, now a nationally known deli with awards from *Bon Appetit*, *Saveur*, and the *Food Network*. (President Obama even ate there on a trip to Michigan in 2014.) I usually got the grilled three-cheese sandwich, which was a huge pile of melted cheese between enormous slices of grilled homemade bread.

We also sometimes cooked together—simple things like pasta or chips and guacamole. And most Sunday mornings we set up a big platter of brunch food: sliced bagels, various cheeses and meats, sliced onions, tomatoes, and lettuce, mustard, and mayonnaise on the side. We would spend the day reading the *New York Times* and noshing on our platter. In the evening, we would have a beer or some wine with dinner. Michael had a relaxed but controlled attitude around food—he never overate—and he had a similar control over substance use. When we were together, I never smoked or did drugs, and we very rarely got drunk. I relied on Michael and Yo's stability during those two years as a grad student to guide me in how much to eat, drink, and consume.

After I finished school I was given one job offer at IBM just outside Washington, DC. The pay was good, and I had always wanted to live in an urban environment. Michael applied for graduate school at the University of Maryland and we moved to DC together, but I lived downtown and he was living forty-five minutes away in Maryland. He wasn't ready to commit to our relationship, so when we arrived we agreed that we would break up.

I rented an apartment near Dupont Circle in DC and commuted by bus more than an hour to IBM. Literally everyone I worked with lived near IBM, so I knew no one downtown. Some days I walked to the Metro crying, feeling lonely and groundless. Without my old friends or many new friends, and finding myself alone every evening, I fell back into unhealthy eating habits. On a typical day I ate a bagel with cream cheese for breakfast, a fried chicken sandwich for lunch, chips or M&M's for an afternoon snack, and toast with pizza sauce and melted cheese for dinner. Focused on my weight, I ran or did aerobics most days after work and continued to fill my body with processed, sugary, and fried foods, and I still binged whenever I was sad.

Still, because of what I'd learned from Yo and Michael, I was at least sitting down for meals now and then. Sometimes I even noticed how food looked and tasted, and once in a while I enjoyed it. One day while waiting in line at the company's cafeteria, I met another young woman. We didn't work in the same department, but we had seen each other in the building. I was intrigued when she led our conversation into territory that most people avoided because of its potential for emotional vulnerability. She asked whether I had siblings, and if so, what my "role" in the family was. Was I the "pretty one," the "smart one," or the "problem child"? She asked how I felt about working at IBM. Was I happy? She was genuinely interested in my answers.

We sat down to eat together. She didn't talk about what she should or shouldn't be eating; she just ate what she wanted and enjoyed it. I was fascinated. Her comfort with emotions and food, the very things that I was most afraid of, was a beacon toward which I wanted to steer my boat. With that meal, Deidre and I began a lifelong friendship that still continues to explore sensitive areas of emotions and spirituality even to this day.

One morning, as I was having breakfast at the bagel shop around the corner from my apartment, I noticed a handsome stranger going into the café.

I was twenty-three at the time. When he came back out, he sat down across from me, introduced himself as Paul, and asked what part of Michigan I was from. I didn't understand how he could know I was from Michigan, but later I found out that he had a second-floor condo with a bay window just across the street from my first-floor apartment and he had seen my parents coming to visit me in a car with Michigan plates. I thought Paul was cute and charming, and I was intrigued when a local character—a scraggly artist named Gardner—stopped by our table to say hello to Paul.

Paul invited me to his apartment to see one of Gardner's paintings and have homemade cheese fondue a few nights later. He claimed to have a secret recipe that had been handed down through the generations, and was so possessive of the recipe that he kept it hidden in his shirt pocket whenever he wasn't reading it. Once the cheese was bubbling, we tore up pieces of French bread, sat on the couch in front of his tiny fireplace, and dipped and ate until all the cheese was gone. He served an ancient white wine stolen from an ex-girlfriend's father's wine cellar. Paul was a dramatic character who moaned with pleasure when he took his first bite of the top-secret fondue. For the first time since I was a child, I was openly celebrating the sensual tastes and smells of a meal.

After a little more than a year, I left IBM and Paul and I became engaged. After Paul and I moved in together, I took a job at Oracle, whose goal was to double in size every year. My first Oracle position involved teaching and consulting, and it meant a lot of travel. Our team worked long hours, and then drank to excess to cope with the pressure. Sometimes we did drugs. This job was definitely more fun, but also much more frenetic, and it fed into my tendency to extremes.

Seeking a way to deal with my stress besides eating, drinking, and doing drugs, and looking for the ease of my early experiences with meditation, I decided to start going to church again. There was a wonderful big, old, urban Presbyterian church near our apartment, which had a focus on social justice issues and being a welcoming community, and I found some respite during the quiet services there.

The Baby Cure

Paul and I got married, and soon I was pregnant. This time, I felt like I had the partner and, hopefully, the inner resources I needed to be a parent. I was excited, and being pregnant was a license to binge without any guilt, be it an entire bag of grapefruit, steak fries of a certain diameter, and most especially, red meat. I gained so much weight during the first trimester that my doctor was convinced I had gestational diabetes until I took the test.

Lucile was born by emergency C-section, after hours of labor and the doctor putting nearly his whole arm inside me to try to turn her around. That was not fun. I had planned for a completely natural birth, but because I hadn't had an epidural, I had to be put under general sedation for the C-section. I wanted to be the mom who objected vehemently to medical interventions, but the pain was so great that I was secretly celebrating going under. I thought, "Please, just hit me over the head with a lead pipe. Just make the pain to go away." Then, immediately, I felt guilty about wanting to be unconscious.

When I woke up, the nurse was holding our beautiful, hairy baby girl in her arms and asked if I wanted to hold her. I was too tired from the sedation, so once I'd confirmed that she was healthy, I fell back asleep. I woke up famished and in the throes of another guilt attack. I couldn't believe that I had been too tired to hold my own baby. Where had she been while I slept it off? Starving and alone in a bassinet?

I was starving too. Our friend Ted showed up with a small brown paper bag. Inside was the most delicious toasted poppy seed bagel with cream cheese I had ever tasted, and I wolfed it down before the nurses brought Lucile into my room. I was thrilled to be finally holding and nursing her, though I still felt guilty about not being awake enough to hold her after her delivery.

Lucile's birth was the first of many times when parenting guilt would sidetrack me from living in the moment. I blamed myself for everything that she experienced, from her allergies (apparently if you don't go through the birth canal you miss a lot of great microbes that can protect you from them) to her later struggles with addiction and eating. I told myself that it must be my genetics, my own compulsive eating, or just my screwed-up parenting. Later I learned that the Buddha had an expression for this and our many other ways of avoiding the direct experience of our suffering—he called it "shooting ourselves with the second arrow."

The Second Arrow

The Buddha told a story about a man who is struck by an arrow and then is immediately struck by another arrow, so that he has both the initial pain of the first wound and the multiplied pain caused by the second arrow. You can think of the first arrow as the external difficulties that arise in our lives over which we have absolutely no control, things such as breaking an arm, being raised by unskillful parents, having a difficult boss, or seeing our children in distress.

The second arrow is the one we shoot with our own minds. By reaching for the wine bottle, the painkillers, or the cheesecake, we cause ourselves additional pain in our attempt to escape the pain of the first arrow. In the moment, it seems like a great idea to eat or drink our troubles away, but even two thousand five hundred years ago, the Buddha knew it wouldn't bring us the happiness and peace that we really need.

Although my position at Oracle was quite intense and involved a lot of travel, I went back to work immediately after delivering Lucile. Having grown up with a highly focused working mother, I told people, "It would be way too boring for me to stay home. What would I do all day?" I hired an elderly woman named Virginia to take care of Lucile and headed back to sell software.

I was sad leaving Lucile after just six weeks, but my denial mechanism was working well, and I got right back into the swing. Just nine months later, Paul and I decided to have a second baby so Lucile would have a sibling to play with while we were both at work.

During my second pregnancy, I craved my usual steak fries, but also a particular thin-crust pizza—the kind I had eaten one time at Barone's in the Chicago suburb of Glen Ellyn—and big juicy ribs. I couldn't get the pizza, so I balanced it out with more ribs. I was an aspiring vegetarian at this point, but my meat cravings were stronger than my commitment to non-harming. Paul surprised me one morning when he looked at me and said, "I think you are having twins." Other than my mother and his mother both being twins, there was no other reason to believe that would be true. But he was right.

I was worried about having two more babies. For one thing, we had just finished renovating our house in a gentrifying neighborhood of the city. I had recently had to carry Lucile around a police situation in front of our house in which there was a suspect lying on the ground and with two police officers pointing their guns at him. I felt I could manage the neighborhood with one baby, but three? Paul was sweet, but he wasn't a huge help with the babies. I wondered how I would manage three babies and my full-time job, which was now a lucrative but very demanding sales position. Paul, fresh from law school, found a low-paying job working for an art lawyer, so the pressure was on me to support the family financially.

My twin pregnancy was normal, other than the doctor-ordered bed rest, which consisted of me taking care of Lucile in the morning, eating whatever my hugely pregnant self wanted to eat, and lying on the couch watching soap operas all afternoon while she napped. No selling software that I didn't care about, no pretending to want to win at any cost, but still receiving my full salary. I was surprised to discover that I wasn't bored at all. (Okay, so maybe I'm forgetting the poop explosions and tedious hours playing with Fisher-Price Little People and animal puppets.)

I went into labor at thirty-seven weeks, and when Doctor Kowalski came into my hospital room to tell me it was time to push the girls out, I didn't want to leave my room because *General Hospital* was just starting and I wanted to watch it. I was in a great mood, excited about having twins, and not yet guilty about destroying Lucile's perfect life as an only child. That came later. Jamie and Veronica were born thirty minutes later, just nineteen minutes apart, without any medical intervention.

I began a part-time work-from-home writing job for Oracle. The financial burden was heavy and we had just bought a new house. But we agreed that my sanity was worth it.

I was now responsible for the nutritional needs of three little girls, and I desperately didn't want to pass on any of my own food craziness to my daughters. Though Paul was there, he deferred to me on most parenting decisions and almost anything related to food. He moved to a new, more demanding but better paying job and we had an unspoken agreement that his role was to be the breadwinner and I was the bread maker. We both had been raised by strong mothers, but both of our mothers had also been the primary caregivers and cooks. We followed a similar model. He came home just in time—well, actually late—for dinner every night, and I did my own work, took care of the girls, and pulled something together for dinner most nights.

I read every parenting book I could find and asked for guidance from the universe. In front of the kids, I acted nonchalant around food, saying and doing the things I thought seemed the most normal, but meanwhile still secretly filling up on carbs and sweets at every opportunity.

I thought that if I didn't acknowledge or talk about my continuing struggle with food, it wouldn't exist and it wouldn't get passed on to our kids. It didn't work. I provided our kids with the very healthiest organic foods we could afford, I kept sugary and processed foods out of the house, and I acted the way I thought a normal person would act around food, and still some of our kids became compulsive about eating. Not all of them, and certainly not all the time, but food addiction was a time bomb just waiting to go off in my perfect little babies.

I worried about them from the time they were very small. They adored sweets, especially Lucile, but I told myself that all kids were like this—and many are. Lucile was the smallest in her class but could finish five cups of juice during snack time. Veronica cried and needed holding and comfort, and because I didn't have a lot of patience, I often resorted to consoling her with snacks. Jamie was quiet, so we called her "the easy one."

I wanted to control their food choices, but not to the point where they wouldn't be able to eat at other kids' houses or go out to dinner. I flip-flopped from day to day. One day I wouldn't allow any sweets, and the next day we would bake two dozen chocolate-chip cookies together. I can see now how much my inconsistency and lack of ease with food helped water their seeds of disordered eating.

I don't think there is one particular thing I could have done that would have prevented my children from their own suffering, but I think our family would have benefited from some open dialogue about food and its challenges. Rather than falling into my old habit of restricting and bingeing—making some foods "good" and others "bad"—I wish we'd had more of an ongoing conversation. All the stories in my mind about food and weight got in the way of having that open conversation. Like my mom, I believed that if we didn't talk about it, it wouldn't happen.

There was still more parenting chaos yet to come. When the twins were about nine months old and Lucile was just two, we were driving back from a puppet show, and a song about homelessness came on the radio. I can't remember the song now, but I began to cry, and cry, and cry. The song was sad, but it was still just a song. The only other time I had been that sensitive was when I was pregnant. But now I was still nursing the twins, and Paul and I hadn't had unprotected sex. I decided to stop at the pharmacy to pick up a pregnancy test just to put my mind at rest. I brought it home, peed on the stick, and set it on the kitchen counter. Paul and I watched the little line go from negative to positive. Neither one of us spoke. We had a two-year-old and two nine-month-olds. Because I was doing technical writing from home, we had lost most of my income. We had just purchased a bigger and more expensive house. And now I was pregnant with our fourth child.

This period of my life is a blur of feeding babies, changing diapers, and working whenever I could find a moment. A highlight was the time Paul and I went with a group of political friends to Bill Clinton's inaugural ball when I was eight months pregnant with our fourth. A week later, in January of 1993, I delivered our first boy, Louie, while Paul ate a Listrani's pepperoni pizza (delivered to the birthing room) and watched the Super Bowl.

I felt overwhelmed by the responsibility of having four little children, and trapped by my inability to leave the house with all of them while Paul was at work. I had to use a triple stroller and a backpack to go grocery shopping or even walk around the block. They ate all day long, so I did too. I was slow to lose the pregnancy weight because I ate their leftovers along with my own meals. I was happy to be a mom and thrilled to have healthy kids, and I was also sad about losing my personal space and my self-determination by having four children in just thirty-seven months.

To allow me a little more freedom, we decided to splurge on hosting an eighteen-year-old au pair from Ireland. While she was inexperienced and young, having Brigid living with us at least allowed me to get out of the house to exercise now and then and to grocery shop without all four kids. It also gave me a bit more time to reflect on my life.

For the first time that I could remember, I felt like I could stop the forward progression of my life. I had reached all the milestones that my family and society expected of me (college degree, marriage, good job, children, house) and I was in a safe and mostly comfortable relationship. I felt I could stop running after something else and be still. I could ask myself questions like, "What's important?" and "What kind of person/parent do I want to be?"

As I would learn later, in order to be mindful of the present moment, we first have to know how to stop. When I began working from home part-time and taking care of babies, I had the chance to slow down. I sat still and quiet while nursing and rocking them, and when they were a little older, I walked at their pace up to the park. If I wanted to connect with my kids, I had to slow down.

And by slowing down, I began to see my life more clearly. I noticed my compulsiveness, especially around food. I saw how I made myself miserable by worrying and obsessing about what I did or didn't do, what I said or didn't say, what I ate or didn't eat, and that I never felt like I fit in anywhere. Noticing these unhealthy ways of thinking didn't make them go away, but once they were out in the open, the landscape of my mind started to change. I couldn't ignore them anymore and I became aware of a desire to transform these habits, so I could enjoy the wonderful life that I had worked so hard to create.

Yo's Dumplings

These are the dumplings that helped me relearn how to enjoy food. Yo made his Chin family recipe for us in his one-bedroom apartment across the hall from mine when we were in graduate school together at the University of Michigan. They are time-consuming, but that's all part of the process. It gave us more time to hang out together in the kitchen. Learning how to be patient in preparing and eating food was something I eventually learned, but I had difficulty back then. When he comes to visit us in DC, we sometimes coerce him into making them with our whole family.

INGREDIENTS:

dumpling skins, either buy at the store (a package of approximately 50 skins)

OR make by hand as follows (check out FoodTube videos for tips on making):

3 cups flour

1 cup hot tap water

½ teaspoon of salt

INGREDIENTS, DIPPING SAUCE:

½ cup soy sauce

¼ cup rice vinegar

¼ cup toasted sesame oil

METHOD, DIPPING SAUCE:

Mix all three ingredients together with a fork or whisk.

(continues)

METHOD, SKINS:

Add the flour to a mixing bowl and add the water.

Mix by hand or in a food processor.

Let rest from 30 minutes to 2 hours, until dough is smooth and pliable.

Divide in half and roll out a rope length.

Split into small walnut size balls and flatten.

Roll into discs using a rolling pin, approximately 3 inches in diameter.

INGREDIENTS, FILLING:

- 7- to 8-ounce package of spiced or flavored firm tofu. Five Spice or Teriyaki works well. Plain is fine if you can't find spiced. Drain the water from the package, then press the tofu with a heavy plate or squeeze it between paper towels to get rid of all the excess water.
- 3 to 4 Napa cabbage leaves, large outer ones
- 4 ounces of Chinese garlic chives, or regular chives if you can't find the Chinese ones
- 4 to 5 shiitake mushrooms
- 2 eggs, beaten
- 2 slices fresh ginger
- 2 cloves garlic
- 1 tablespoon soy sauce
- 1 tablespoon sesame oil
- 3 tablespoons canola oil

METHOD, FILLING:

Finely julienne the cabbage leaves.

Chop the chives into tiny pieces.

Chop the tofu and mushrooms into small pieces.

Mince the garlic and ginger.

Heat 1 tablespoon canola oil in a nonstick wok, and add the ginger and garlic.

Add the remaining ingredients and sauté until the vegetables wilt and the mix dries somewhat.

Add the beaten eggs and soy sauce, and just barely cook (eggs are the binder).

Transfer to a bowl, add sesame oil, mix, and let cool.

Add 1 heaping teaspoon of filling to each dumpling skin, leaving enough dough to enclose the dumpling.

Pleat the dumpling (refer to the FoodTube video), or simply pinch the skin closed, pierogi-style.

Set it aside on a floured surface, and repeat until all the skins are filled.

Heat the remaining oil, and add the dumplings in batches to cook.

Let dumplings cook until bottoms are lightly browned.

Add 1 cup water and cover.

Cook over high to medium-high heat until most of the water evaporates.

Remove cover and let the remaining water evaporate.

Carefully use a spatula to release the dumplings, and turn off the burner.

Serve with dipping sauce.

Makes approximately 40 dumplings.

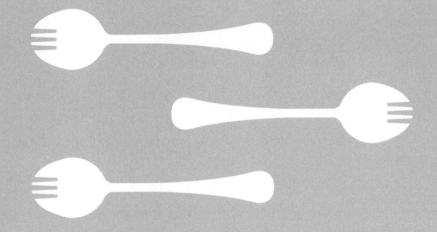

3.

SLICING, DICING, SAUTÉING, and BURNING

More and more I have come to admire resilience. Not the simple resistance of a pillow, whose foam returns over and over to the same shape, but the sinuous tenacity of a tree: finding the light newly blocked on one side, it turns to another.

—JANE HIRSHFIELD, "OPTIMISM"

I'm a senior in high school, and my sister Maggie and I are on a clothes shopping trip in the quaint upscale Detroit suburb of Birmingham, which is filled with cute boutiques and cafés. We are having lunch at Olga's Kitchen, a tiny dumpy Greek restaurant in one of the shopping arcades. We each order a greasy gyro covered with freshly chopped tomatoes, onions, and a creamy yogurt sauce. It comes wrapped in something called "Olga Bread" that tastes like a cross between pita bread and a sweet pancake.

Behind the counter, as in Greece, pressed lamb is spinning on a spit. It's crowded and there are no more than four small tables along the arcade wall. We grab a table and wait for our order. When they call my sister's name, she picks up our gyros with two feta salads and a side of curly fries and brings them to the table. This is an unusual outing for the two of us. We almost never go out together. It feels almost unreal because of its rarity. I eat and talk nonstop in order to control my discomfort with the intimacy—I think my sister will find me stupid or embarrassing. The sweet, savory, and greasy food is comforting, and eating it calms my hyperaroused nervous system.

I NEVER MET OLGA HERSELF, but I developed a lifelong obsession with Olga's Kitchen food. I don't know if it was my Armenian heritage, the sweet bread, or just my taste buds, but I could never get enough of their gyros. I liked the lamb gyro, but I also loved the three-cheese version, and later I discovered the fresh-vegetable Olga.

I ate Olga's in college, even when I had to write bad checks to get it. Olga's food comforted me when I was down. When I broke up with a boy, failed a test, or was worried about something, I ate at Olga's. I thought that if I could just get to Olga's, I'd be okay. Much of the food was supersalty, cheesy, and processed, but like any addict, I didn't care. When I moved to DC, I found an Olga's Kitchen thirty minutes from my house, and I was eating there when my water broke with Louie.

When I sat down with a gyro, for a single moment I didn't need anything else. Dr. Gabor Maté, author of *In the Realm of Hungry Ghosts: Close Encounters with Addiction* and longtime addictions counselor, describes this moment: "The fundamental addiction is to the fleeting experience of not being addicted. The addict craves the absence of the craving state. For a brief moment he's liberated from emptiness, from boredom, from lack of meaning, from yearning, from being driven, or from pain."

Suffering Happens

Thinking about and eating food was, and sometimes still is, a distraction from my inner mean girl—the voice that I first heard when I rejected the compliment about my orange dress. Its underlying refrain is, "You're ugly and fat, and no one likes you." Tying up my mind in knots around food obsessions—avoidance and cravings—and fears about my weight drowned out the mean voice to a manageable level. It wasn't until my mind began to settle as a result of meditation that I could learn to hear that critical voice without believing its story.

I didn't yet know why I was driven to such craziness around food—craving, bingeing, purging, and starving myself. I just knew these things made me feel better for a moment, though later I always felt worse. I couldn't see that my dissatisfaction was caused by habits of thinking rooted in both my genetics and in a childish and unsustainable belief that I could avoid any pain by keeping myself distracted with food and body image.

One of the Buddha's first teachings was the Four Noble Truths. The First Noble Truth is that pain is a part of everyone's life. We are all going to experience difficulties, from something as devastating as a cancer diagnosis to something as common as unrequited love. No matter how hard we try, we can't avoid it.

The Second Noble Truth is the causes of our suffering isn't just the situations we experience. What really keeps us tormented are the cravings, aversions, and obsessions that we use to avoid feeling our pain—the second arrow we shoot at ourselves. All my addictions and eating dysfunctions were ways of avoiding the underlying pain that arises in my life.

We aren't comfortable with the unpleasant parts of life and so we do anything and everything to avoid them and hang on to what we consider pleasant. When we get the thing we must have or avoid the thing we are afraid of, we experience a moment of non-craving. We eat three pieces of delicious cheesecake and feel temporarily satiated. But because nothing is permanent, including pleasant feelings, eventually we feel dissatisfied (and hangry) again. What we are really after is a deeper, longer-lasting peace. I call that kind of peace contentment. I think it's what Christians refer to as "the peace of God, which surpasses all understanding."

The Third Noble Truth is that it is possible to find that contentment, even in the midst of our ever-changing feelings and experiences. The Fourth Noble Truth is the Buddha's prescription for finding contentment, which he called the Eightfold Path. I describe the Eightfold Path more fully in chapter 8, but an essential part of the path is the practice of mindfulness meditation.

I had touched on contentment by doing self-hypnosis as a teenager and by sitting in the silent church as a young adult. But sometimes I confused the moment of non-craving (having the gyro in my mouth, or being hyped up on cocaine) with contentment, which is like confusing a plastic dog-chew carrot with a real carrot pulled from the earth. You might initially think the dog chew is a real carrot, but only until you touch or taste it. Each time I got an Olga's gyro (or a drink, or some drugs, or whatever) I had the momentary sense that this dog chew was a real carrot. Only later, after the food and drugs wore off, did I recognize that I had been fooled again. Once I began to meditate regularly, I knew experientially what inner contentment, and real carrots, tasted like.

Searching in the Dark

One of the foundations for peace of mind during my parenting years was movement. I went to aerobics or yoga classes almost every day, and when I couldn't do that, I would go for a short run. This was helpful. But I still longed for something deeper—a spiritual path. I had started taking yoga during my second pregnancy and loved it. I was drawn to the meditative way we moved our bodies, but I was occasionally put off by the "woo-woo" qualities of some of the classes I attended.

I wasn't really searching for something outside of myself, like God, Shiva, or Brahma; I merely wanted a way of living that would calm my compulsive and somewhat unstable mind. Paul and I encouraged each other's creative aspects, but neither of us had much stability, and we laughed, fought, ate, and partied to excess. We pushed the edges. We had the most outrageous kids' birthday parties (when Batman and Robin staged a fight in our living room, some of the three-year-old boys ran upstairs in tears)—nothing was done in moderation, including eating. Food was one way to create a sense of grounding, so I beelined for the kitchen whenever I was stressed.

I loved books, and I often took the kids to events at the library and the local bookstore. While there I would scan the books about yoga and meditation, sometimes buying one. In one book I learned about mantras (repeating certain words over and over), being aware of my breathing, concentrating on an object, and something called Bubble Meditation, in which you envision your thoughts being encapsulated by bubbles and floating away. I still didn't know anyone else who practiced meditation. I tried one thing after another without consistency, but with a lot of curiosity and hope.

One of the books I found was Starhawk's *The Fifth Sacred Thing*, which propelled me to look for a Wiccan group. The one I found met in an empty storefront in Silver Spring, Maryland, a kind of pop-up coven. At our meetings we learned spells—recipes for everything from healing illnesses to finding love. After only a few weeks, the seriousness became too much for me, and I dropped out of the coven. The only thing that stuck with me from the coven was the fundamental Wiccan creed "Harm None," which I felt was a reasonable summation of any spiritual pursuit.

Exploring these various avenues was like going to a wine or chocolate tasting. I started to find out which practices made me feel better and which annoyed me. Practices based on real-life transformation and personal growth, not on dogma, tasted best to me. The fact that I was the primary caregiver of four very young kids limited the amount of time I could commit to participating in anything, especially if children were not part of the process. Unfortunately, meditation books rarely, if ever, mentioned children. Based on my reading, it seemed that everyone practicing meditation (and even yoga) were single people with no kids and no job.

Our house was insane. In just three years we had gone from newlyweds to a family with four babies, two dogs, a cat, two parents, and Brigid, who was in some ways more like a fifth child than a nanny. Paul had to work longer hours to make up for my reduced income, the au pair salary, and our four dependents. He was rarely home for dinner and literally worked through the night once a week to get caught up. One day I stopped at the ATM to get money for the grocery store, and the IRS had emptied our account because we were so far behind in our taxes. Eventually we were able to repay our debts by reaching out to Paul's extended family. Someone was always sick, we never got enough sleep, and I was sure most of our troubles were somehow my fault.

As I dove more deeply into meditation and yoga, I decided to commit to becoming a vegetarian in the hopes of reducing the suffering of all sentient beings. Paul kept eating meat. We disagreed on what to feed the kids, but I convinced him to let me try raising them vegetarian. On a cross-country drive when Lucile was only five, we stopped at a McDonald's to use the restroom. While I was tending to the other kids, Lucile asked her dad to buy her a burger. She gulped it down and begged for another. She ate the second one, and still wanted more. Two and a half hamburgers later, Paul convinced me that she might have nutritional needs that weren't being met by her veggie diet. After that, we let the kids decide if they wanted meat.

They usually did, so most nights I cooked meat for them and vegetarian for me—just like my mother had done for all those years.

Pass the Parenting Guilt

Throughout my early parenting days, I continued to worry that I would repeat the compulsive patterns of my childhood and cause my own children to be afraid of food like I was. Implicit in that fear was the belief that my parents had caused all my eating problems and, naturally, that I was to blame for all of my children's suffering. I don't believe that now, but I did then. So I was always looking for ways to be a good parent, to do it right. I would have given anything to keep my children from developing that inner voice of self-loathing that had made me chronically depressed and guilty for decades. I thought that there was a right way to parent, and if I found it, none of us would suffer. Marshall Rosenberg, author of *Nonviolent Communication (NVC): A Language of Life*, says, "Hell is having children and thinking there's such a thing as a good parent."

When my kids were sick or in pain, I panicked. Lucile started having chronic diarrhea, urinary infections, and rashes when she was still a baby. We had her tested for about five million diseases, none of which she had. She cried when she started kindergarten and then developed daily headaches, which turned out to be a case of mononucleosis, something unusual in a child that young.

The day after she was born, Jamie turned yellow with newborn jaundice and had to be kept under bilirubin lights, and I spent every minute of her stay bothering the doctors until they finally decided she could go home after just a few hours. Veronica needed extra holding and comforting, and developed several serious phobias that required a lot of attention. In every situation, I wanted to keep them from feeling pain. Seeing them suffer was the first arrow. When I wasn't able to prevent that, I shot myself with the second arrow of guilt, overeating, or getting drunk.

One day, when Jamie was four, I noticed that her right eye didn't seem to be tracking with her left, so I took her to see the pediatrician. The doctor wasn't convinced, but he offered to give Jamie an eye exam.

Jamie and I stood in the hallway. The nurse stood at the other end of the hall holding a deck of cards, each with a different shape printed on it. Before holding up the first card, the nurse asked me to help Jamie cover her left eye with a round piece of paper on a stick. We covered her eye. The nurse held up the first card and asked Jamie what it was. She didn't answer.

The nurse got a little impatient and raised her voice to coax Jamie into answering, but still got no answer. Jamie was usually quiet, but she was also a people-pleaser and always did as she was told. I looked at her to try to figure out why she was stonewalling, and noticed her right eye moving around strangely like it was desperately searching for the shape. I said, "Jamie, can you see the shape?" She shook her head. "Jamie, can you see the nurse?" Again, she shook her head. "Jamie, can you see anything?" As the silent tears began to slide down her cheeks, I understood why she hadn't answered. She was completely blind in her right eye.

We were sent off to see a specialist who confirmed that Jamie had permanent damage in the retina of her right eye and would probably never see anything out of it. The doctor guessed it could have been caused by an eye infection in utero, but they couldn't confirm any definite cause. I dropped Jamie at home and then stopped at the liquor store where I bought a large bottle of Scotch. I drank half the bottle before I could talk to my husband or my parents about what had happened. I didn't want to be conscious of or feel how Jamie might suffer as a result of her disability. I couldn't accept that her suffering was something that I would never be able to control. So, rather than feel it, I checked out.

Meeting the Moment

Around this time, my old friend Deidre suggested that I go on a retreat being held outside Prescott, Arizona, led by the wise cultural anthropologist

Angeles Arrien. Though it wasn't specifically a yoga or meditation retreat, Deidre had been changed by a similar retreat, and she knew I was still looking for some spiritual ground. During the retreat we meditated, created and sang a self-empowerment song (mine was "I Am Annie," set to the tune of "I Am Woman," which I never had the confidence to sing), and went on drumming journeys. I alternated between thinking the whole week was ridiculous and wishing I could really join in. Connecting with other people in such a vulnerable way was exhilarating and also scary as hell. Other than Deidre, most of the people I knew well seemed sarcastic, cynical, or tightly wound. I realized later that maybe that was just my own reflection.

In Arizona, I touched into the ease that I had felt so many years earlier doing self-hypnosis. I experienced moments of quiet in my mind, which I hadn't known were possible. I saw how my mind created stories about other people, the world, and myself, and how so many of these stories, especially the ones about my body and eating, had caused me years of difficulty. I could imagine myself being part of this kind of group again. At home I still reacted in some of the same ways—eating and drinking to avoid feeling—but inside I knew that something else was possible and that I was on my way there. I didn't yet know what form it would take, but I knew I wanted to find a practice that included spiritual and contemplative elements without any dogma.

I wanted to be guided by the values I could feel inside me whenever I sat still, not by my neurotic fear of intimacy and my constant inner judgments. Could I hear my neurotic mind without believing the content? On my flight back to DC from Arizona, I connected wholeheartedly with the man sitting next to me, even though he was a socially awkward talker and seemed desperate for company. In the past I would have either pretended to be "nice" and then later created a funny story about him to entertain my sister, or been just bitchy enough to prevent him from engaging. I would have felt both superior and ashamed of my actions. This time, without much effort, I felt genuine kindness toward him, and didn't spin out into judgments of him or me.

This was a novel experience and a skill I hoped to expand upon for my own sake and for my children's. I had brought home with me a close-up photo I had taken of a desert plant to remind me of what it felt like to stop and look at something deeply rather than always racing past. When I got home I posted the photo in my kitchen, and whenever I looked at it I remembered my intention to slow down and be there.

But my post-retreat high didn't last too long. Like every family, we continued to face difficulties that I didn't know how to handle, though we loved each other intensely and had a lot of fun together. My general dissatisfaction continued, but now at least I had some ideas about where to turn. I bought and read Thich Nhat Hanh's first book, *The Miracle of Mindfulness*. While reading it I became aware that this was the first book that had ever made complete sense to me. Reading it was like someone finally telling me the truth about the way life really is.

One thing that especially struck me was Thich Nhat Hanh's assertion that taking care of ourselves is the best way to take care of others. He said that meditation is not an escape from reality, but a way to dive deeper into reality. This was important because I didn't want to find another escape route, and I didn't want to focus just on myself and abandon my family. I wanted to learn to live wholeheartedly and include all parts of my life. But I had to start by getting to know myself.

As I began to practice meditation more regularly, a very unpleasant piece of reality began to surface. The repressed memory of the abortion I had at eighteen started showing up in my mind. Some part of me knew it was true and didn't want to stuff it back down, so I decided to try something new. Rather than denying the memory and associated feelings of guilt and shame that were arising, I would face them directly and with compassion for myself. I had never been to therapy, but I instinctively felt this was something I couldn't do on my own. I found a psychotherapist who specialized in helping women who'd gotten abortions. Together she and I watched as the deep feelings of grief, shame, and regret arose, were embraced, and slowly settled back into position as simply another memory—a sad memory, but just a memory. My experiment had been successful, and I began to trust my feelings a little bit more.

During an unusually warm fall, we took a weekend trip to Chesapeake Bay with several other families. One of the couples got into a fight. Another of the women gave them some advice, which created more animosity among the group. I knew it would blow over, but I felt anxious and vulnerable, and I wanted to escape. We were on a remote beach on the Eastern Shore, however, and I was responsible for making and serving the dinner for our ten collective children that evening. By the time the kids finished dinner, I had made my escape into an entire bottle of red wine. I was wasted.

Tensions were still high as the adults put their kids to bed and then sat down to eat their own dinner. Although I was already drunk, I continued to pour myself more wine and ate several helpings of mashed potatoes. I wasn't the only one drinking, but I felt alone. After dinner, the bickering continued and someone unwisely suggested we get high.

Just before midnight, we jumped into canoes and rowed out into the bay, leaving our children, ages ten and under, sleeping in cabins by the water, alone. I don't remember anything that happened after dinner. The next thing I do remember was waking up in physical and emotional pain, sick from all the food and wine, and stumbling into the bathroom to face myself in the mirror, leaving Paul sleeping it off in bed. I was drowning in shame. In the mirror I saw a mother who was so afraid of her feelings that she chose to binge eat, get blackout drunk, and leave her kids alone on a remote beach at night rather than simply sitting with how she felt.

This was it for me. I didn't know how my life would change, but I knew it had to. I promised myself that this would be the last time I would get smashed. And it was.

Finding Friends

Not too much later that summer, a catalog arrived in the mail from the Omega Institute, a retreat and conference center in upstate New York. I sat down and read through the catalog page by page, dreaming about the retreats and programs, any one of which I would have loved to attend—yoga trainings, meditation workshops, and sweat lodges. In the centerfold was a two-page spread describing a five-day retreat in the fall with Thich Nhat Hanh. I was intrigued, but I didn't think it would be possible to leave Paul with the kids for a week during the school year.

Then, toward the bottom of the page I saw a note that changed everything: "Families welcome. Programs for children ages six and up." Louie was six, the twins were eight, and Lucile was nine. The price was very reasonable. Not only could I learn and practice mindfulness with the Zen master Thich Nhat Hanh, whose books were the basis for everything I understood at that point about mindfulness and meditation, but my children would be able to learn alongside me. There would be three meals a day that I wouldn't have to cook or clean up, and half of each day would be spent in silence. It sounded amazing. I knew Paul wouldn't want to join us, but I asked him anyway. He said he would rather work. I wasn't surprised, and was even a bit relieved to know that I wouldn't have to try to convince him to try something new; I could focus on myself and my kids. Within a week, we had registered for the retreat.

October finally arrived, and I loaded all four kids into our old black Volvo wagon, and we headed up to Rhinebeck, New York, for our first mindfulness retreat. I had no idea what to expect, but I hoped that this mindfulness practice would transform my habitual patterns of suppressing and avoiding my life through using food and other addictions.

At the retreat, the five of us were provided a ten-foot by twelve-foot room almost entirely taken up by two twin beds, and we shared a bathroom with the single woman next door. We arrived late on the first evening and, though we hadn't had time to stop for dinner, we dropped our bags in the room and went straight to the orientation talk with Thich Nhat Hanh, leaving our shoes outside the door with hundreds of other pairs.

Families were instructed to sit at the front of the enormous meditation hall, packed wall to wall with mindfulness practitioners. I wrangled my hangry gang up toward the front of the hall, squeezed into the third row, and sat down with all four kids crawling around and on top of me, begging me for food.

A few minutes into Thich Nhat Hanh's talk, Lucile opened my purse and took out the key to our room. She whispered, "I'm leaving!" and headed out through the ocean of people. I couldn't chase after her because of the other three children hanging from my body, the silent crowd around me, and the fact that Thich Nhat Hanh was speaking only a few feet in front of us. I couldn't scream my usual, "Get back here!" or leap up and run after her. My face must have reflected my terror because a compassionate woman gently collared Lucile and brought her back to me. I was relieved and surprised by the kindness I experienced that night and all throughout the week.

We ate the delicious, vegetarian meals in semi-silence at a table with the few other families who were there. For breakfast we had oatmeal, eggs, and toast. I discovered the rich world of nut butters and nut milks; they served almond, cashew, and peanut butter in addition to tahini, which I had never eaten outside of hummus. We were offered soy, almond, or rice milk to add to our oatmeal or herbal tea. I was in heaven. For lunch we had broccoli-tofu stir-fry, vegan crab cakes, and a burrito bar; and for dinner there were dishes like vegetarian chili, spinach pie, and baked ziti.

During the long mornings listening to talks and meditating, I thought about lunch. In the afternoons, while halfway participating in the small discussion groups or supporting the children's program, I thought about dinner. We were taught that we should slow down our eating, chew each bite at least thirty times, and pay attention to the sensations arising while we ate. It was difficult for my mind to stay present for more than a few seconds. During meals, I alternated between tasting my food and distracting myself by looking around, reading and rereading the signs posted around the dining room.

On the third morning I found a handwritten note in our shared bathroom from the woman next door. My heart sank when I saw it. I assumed that she was, understandably, annoyed by the crazy, barely-keeping-it-together family next door. Why wouldn't a neat single woman complain about the toothpaste-lined sink or the all-hours whining and fighting over the two beds? Tears of surprise and relief came to my eyes as I read the note. It simply said that she loved having us next door and that hearing the sounds of a family made her smile. I honestly wondered if she was being sarcastic.

That week, I saw how people who practiced mindfulness regularly were different from me. They seemed happier and more peaceful. I wanted to be a person who would scoop up a frantic mother's child and return her without even a hint of judgment. I wanted to know the joy I saw on the faces of the monks and nuns as they played soccer with the children on the lawn. I wanted the ease and patience I saw in the other parents who trusted and were able to give their kids space. I wanted to share about my feelings as fearlessly as others in group discussions. I wanted to slow down enough to taste and enjoy my food. I left that retreat determined to bring the practice home so that I could enjoy each moment of my life and not stay trapped in my sarcastic, judgmental, avoidant mind. My kids were happy to be heading home again, but it seemed they had really enjoyed having time together in such a serene and happy setting.

At the retreat we were invited to receive The Five Mindfulness Trainings. The Five Mindfulness Trainings were explained as guidelines to help us end suffering and create inner and outer peace. (See Appendices on page 233 for extended version.) They seemed easy enough:

1. Revere life, don't kill;
2. Practice generosity, don't steal;
3. Protect integrity, don't engage in sexual misconduct;
4. Use mindful speech and listen to others;
5. Consume in a wholesome way, don't use food to cover up pain, and don't use any intoxicants.

Just as I had jumped at the chance to be born again that long-ago day at the Baptist church, there I was at 6:30 a.m. in front of eight hundred other people promising that I would practice these five trainings to the best of my ability. The first four seemed simple enough. Number five was going to be a challenge. But, after hitting bottom with my alcohol consumption, I was desperate for anything that would help me stop running away from my feelings and just live.

I cried most of the way home from the retreat because I didn't trust myself to follow through. I wanted so much to be free, but I just didn't know if I could do it.

I quit drinking and began to practice meditation as often as I thought of it, once or twice a week. I tried to encourage all of us to pay more attention to the sensations of eating, but my efforts petered out after only a few weeks. It was very difficult to change ingrained habits, and since he hadn't been at the retreat, Paul wasn't as excited as I was about all of my newfangled ideas.

The week after we got home, Lucile drew a picture of the garden and grounds of Omega with flowers and people wandering about. In the foreground was an enormous brick wall, and in front of the wall she had drawn her family. I interpreted it as Lucile feeling like we were outsiders to this happy place, prevented from joining in by an enormous impenetrable wall.

I went back to eating mindlessly and compulsively, especially when I felt stressed. But I had taken a first step. Although no one else could see it, I could feel my attitude toward food beginning to soften. I now believed that a peaceful relationship to food was possible, and that mindfulness was the vehicle that would get me there.

Waking Up

Over the next two years, I found out that I was more reliant on alcohol than I had realized. A few times, especially in settings where I felt socially awkward, I gave in and got a little tipsy. When we had a party or I went to my book group, I drank wine. What I discovered was that I couldn't be mindful at all when I was drinking (or even the next morning). I also found out that I didn't really like the person I was when I was drinking, even though she had gotten me through a lot of uncomfortable social situations.

I woke up every day feeling like I had been run over by a train and could barely drag myself out of bed. I had been using food, alcohol, and drugs to avoid the lonely, angry, and sad parts of myself. As I weaned myself from these addictions, I had to go through a very difficult period of withdrawal. The voices of my inner misery, telling me I was worthless, fat, and alone, got louder. Without the bulletproof glass of my alcohol and food addictions, I was staring unprotected down the barrel of despair. Without a teacher, a community, or a regular meditation practice, it was difficult to stay upright. I went through the motions, but I stopped caring about my life.

And yet, I was so grateful for my family. My children brought me reams of joy, and Paul was always supportive. Most evenings we had a family dinner, and I cooked meat or fish for Paul and the kids and a simple vegetarian option for me. The first mindfulness training had reminded me of my intention not to destroy life, and I took that to mean I should remain a vegetarian. I felt good about not eating meat (though now and then I still craved ribs), and I wanted to get my kids back to a vegetarian diet too, but they all seemed more than happy with meat and potatoes. Although I didn't want to continue to cook meat I wanted them to be happy, so being the dutiful wife and mother, I didn't say anything.

As my low mood turned into depression, I found it hard to maintain any sense of mindful eating. When I was feeling sad, it was difficult to do anything—even shopping for groceries seemed overwhelming—so I overate to quiet the sadness and allow myself to sleep. When I woke up, I was ashamed of myself, and that made me more depressed. I was back in the cycle of numbing then shame, then numbing then shame. I had seen this cycle in my dad, and I knew it in myself. Soon I would see it begin to show up in my precious children.

Each of our kids has had their own relationship with food over the years, and none have been completely smooth. Lucile and Veronica's difficulties were the most dramatic and required the most interventions. Both eventually spent time in residential eating disorder and addiction treatment. But that would come later.

PARALLAX PRESS

Please send in this card to receive a copy of our catalog.
Add your email address to sign up for our monthly newsletter.

Please print

Name _____

Address _____

City _____ State _____ Zip _____

Country _____

Email _____

facebook.com/parallaxpress • parallax.org • twitter.com/parallaxpress

Get the latest news, author updates, and special offers online!

PARALLAX PRESS

P.O. Box 7355

Berkeley, CA 94707

When we attended our second meditation retreat together—this one at the Ascutney Mountain resort in Vermont—I noticed how much my children were opening up. At this retreat, the five of us were housed in a two-bedroom ski condo with nine other people. We were given the living room to ourselves for the week. On the second day, Lucile, usually very reserved, put her arm around me while we walked to the dining hall. Between activities she would sneak up and plant a kiss on my cheek. These kinds of small but loving moments with my children gave me glimpses of the peace and connection that I was craving.

There were only twelve children in the entire retreat, but all four of my kids enjoyed the week and had a blast playing soccer and running down hills with the monks and nuns. The five of us were our own Sangha—a community of practitioners. We were on this journey together, at least for the time being.

In each of the Thich Nhat Hanh retreats I attended, we were invited into groups of twenty to thirty people to meet daily to talk about our practice. On my first few retreats, I was still very mistrusting of the other people. While we sat in a circle, listened to the meditation bell, and took turns sharing, I was silently judging each person. That guy was weird-looking, that woman was "too into it," that woman was annoyingly perfect, that guy was stupid, etc. I categorized each person as either better than, worse than, or equal to me.

All day, I scanned the crowds to determine who was a better or worse meditator than I, who was a better or worse mom than I was, and in the dining hall, instead of focusing on the colors, taste, and smell of my food, I was looking around to see who was a better or worse mindful eater. This "game" kept me living in my head. I stayed disconnected from my senses and isolated myself in my own little world of judgment.

But on these retreats, men and women went out of their way to engage with me. Over the course of each retreat, I would slowly give up my judgmental ways and by the end of the retreat I liked most, if not all, of the people that I met. Over and over, I learned that I didn't have to isolate myself by judging people or comparing myself to them, and that doing so only perpetuated my loneliness.

"I also settled into mindful eating, and by the time each retreat ended, I was eating my food with full awareness, enjoying every bite without my usual obsessive thoughts. I noticed a feeling of space opening up in my mind as I practiced more mindfulness. Anything felt possible. Sometimes I noticed fear too—I wondered what might arise if I let that vast expanse of spaciousness just be there. So, instead of just being with the space, I distracted myself with the second arrow of fear and worry.

At home, without the structure of the retreat, the open space I had cultivated in my mind was overwhelming. As my mind quieted, questions arose about what my purpose in life really was, and did my life really matter? I found myself pondering the Buddhist term "aimlessness" or "desirelessness," which means not seeking happiness by running after things outside of ourselves. But if I wasn't running after something, what was I "supposed to be" doing?

My life was full of wonderful moments—the kids were all healthy and doing well in school. Paul was busy at work but loving it. Even still, I found it hard to be grateful or to focus on positive aspects of my life. I had always run after something—approval, a degree, a life purpose, even happiness. If I had nothing to run after, life seemed meaningless. I was like a dog who had been raised in a puppy mill her whole life—when she is finally let out of her cage, she is afraid of the wide open space.

The thought of not having to run was inconceivable. I started having panic attacks. When I thought about aimlessness, it felt like I was poking at my heart with a fork. There was no way to go back into my cage, and it seemed there was no way to move forward. I briefly thought about ending my life, but I knew I couldn't and wouldn't do that to my kids.

I didn't yet know about the way our minds are hardwired to focus on negative thoughts. I still had to learn that the way to avoid despair was by learning to embrace my negative feelings with compassion and paying closer attention to my positive feelings and memories and creating more of a balance in my body-mind.

Negativity Bias

During one of our first mindfulness retreats, a Buddhist monk told the story of how he learned about negativity bias. This monk had been a child in Vietnam during the war and had seen his home bombed and had feared for his life. He was an extremely intelligent boy and left Vietnam to go to college in Texas. He majored in chemical engineering, and had begun working toward his PhD.

But he wasn't happy. He met a Buddhist teacher and, after much consideration, decided to become a monk. He followed his teacher around night and day, asking him questions about how he should practice. He read voraciously, and would come to his teacher and ask questions about what he was learning. "Tell me why there are the Four Noble Truths. What is the Eightfold Path? How do I get to nirvana?" Each time, his teacher answered with a question, "Dear monk, do you see the beautiful flower there?" or "Can you see all the colors in the sunset?" or "My dear brother, look at the moon this evening, isn't it lovely?"

The monk got more and more agitated with his teacher. He had left his studies and traveled across the world to become a monk, and now he wanted to learn something. He expected to be taught the practice of meditation, not to look at flowers, sunrises, and the moon. Just as he was about to give up and leave the monastery, he suddenly realized what his teacher was trying to do. His teacher was helping the monk to transform his negative way of thinking, his negativity bias, by training him to be able to see the many conditions for happiness that are always available in the present moment.

The negativity bias isn't unique to those who, like the monk, have been through trauma. All humans have a negativity bias that causes us to remember and focus on negative feelings and memories more than positive ones. It makes sense if we think about human evolution. Life was very dangerous for hunters and gatherers; we had to be sure we were safe, so it was better to worry when we didn't need to worry than not worry when we should have been worrying.

Neurobiologist Rick Hanson, author of *Buddha's Brain: The Practical Neuroscience of Happiness, Love, and Wisdom*, says, "Your brain has a built-in negativity bias that primes you for avoidance. This bias makes you suffer in a variety of ways. For starters, it generates an unpleasant background of anxiety, which for some people can be quite intense; anxiety also makes it harder to bring attention inward for self-awareness or contemplative practice, since the brain keeps scanning to make sure there is no problem." He goes on to say that our brains are like Velcro for negative experiences and Teflon for positive ones.

What it means for us today is that we can balance the difficult parts of our lives by training ourselves to pay closer attention to fleeting pleasant moments, like when we see a bright red cardinal land on a leafless tree in the middle of winter. If we don't take those moments to actively encourage joy into our consciousness, negative feelings will dominate our mind. This is what was happening to me. I didn't know how to generate happiness to lighten the despair I was feeling as I began to withdraw from my addiction to food and alcohol.

The comedian Louis C.K. has a hilarious skit that reminds us not to get caught in our habitually negative mind. In response to people who complain about enduring a flight delay at the airport, he says, "Oh really, and what happened next? Did you fly through the air incredibly like a bird? Did you partake in the miracle of human flight? Wow, you're flying! It's amazing!" This moment is simply this moment. And when we can see that our despair is based mostly on transient thoughts and feelings, chances are we can find something pleasant or at least humorous in the moment we are in.

Hungry Ghosts

I cherished my mindfulness practice but wasn't sure if it could really transform the mental pain I was in. I went back to therapy. My therapist was a meditator, so we practiced breathing in and out with the sadness. I cried through most of the hour.

Our family had left the socially-engaged urban church downtown, and we now attended a more upscale Episcopal church, which provided us with comforting words and beautiful music, but where I never made a single personal connection. During the ten minutes between the worship service and the kids' Sunday school, a ten-foot-long table was loaded with box after box of Krispy Kreme donuts—which, to be honest, may have been the reason we kept going for as many years as we did.

I was what Buddhists call a "hungry ghost." In his book, *In the Realm of Hungry Ghosts: Close Encounters with Addiction*, Dr. Gabor Maté defines hungry ghosts as pathetic creatures with "scrawny necks, small mouths, emaciated limbs, and large bloated bellies," whose hunger can never be satisfied. We have this constant aching emptiness because the things we think will fill us up are exactly the things that make us hungrier. Hungry ghosts are out of touch with the very aspects of ourselves that know and tell us what we need: our bodies and our senses.

I decided to go back to graduate school to see if I could find what I needed. I thought if I went to divinity school maybe I would find a God who could help me. Maybe I would become a minister or at least find out how to stop my constant aching emptiness and learn to be more present for my family, my friends, and for my own life. It seemed like an impulsive decision from the outside. But something inside kept pushing me toward divinity school, and the Howard University School of Divinity in particular, so I listened to it. As always, Paul was supportive of my decision. He could see that I was struggling and looking for direction, and he liked the idea of me bringing a more spiritual flavor into our family life.

During my two years at Howard, a historically black university, I learned a whole lot about my own mind—the racist thoughts that I had been conditioned to believe and my one-sided view of Christianity—and I learned how to pray. I didn't know consciously why the only divinity school I wanted to attend was Howard, but once I was there it became clearer. Howard's focus was on liberation theology and social engagement, not on simple theology like most of the other schools. I wanted something that I could apply to my life, not something more to think about. I didn't find comfort in the teachings of Christianity in the way I had hoped. I was disappointed in the Bible, and angry about the violent history of the Christian church. But I did find that I had a strong calling toward spiritual service.

What I valued most was the social justice focus at Howard. For our final exam in New Testament class, we took a bus one evening to a pre-adjudication home for young men who had been arrested but hadn't yet had been to court. The men took turns asking us questions about God and religion. I was the only white person in the house, and likely the only one who practiced Buddhism. I had never been more nervous for a test. I wanted to give a strong confident answer about God that would encourage these boys to find their own spiritual path, but not come off as arrogant or say something too far outside their Christian comfort zone for them to relate to.

One by one, my classmates were asked questions about Jesus, God, and the church. They testified to being saved, shared their histories of struggle and discrimination, and their love of the church. Finally a young man pointed to me and asked, "You. Is there only one God?" This question came as a relief to me because it wasn't about church dogma.

I said that there was indeed only one God but it was called by many names. I listed some of the different names God has been called and how there is very little real difference between the aims of the major religions. This moment helped crystallize my understanding of what I really needed to heal. As much as I tried, I couldn't cultivate the BFF relationship with Jesus that so many of my classmates spoke about, and I spent every worship service translating the liturgy into mindfulness language. This realization helped me accept the reality that I wasn't cut out for Christian ministry, and maybe not even for church. I graduated and immediately signed up for another mindfulness retreat.

With my deepening commitment to the practice of mindfulness and my relationships with other spiritual seekers, I was gaining confidence in my path, which included regular yoga, meditation, meditation groups (Sangha), and less often church. I was finally able to let go of my reliance on intoxicants and was transforming my food addiction, but underneath was a lot of accumulated tenderness and unhappiness that needed my care. Author and American Buddhist nun Pema Chödrön says, "This continual ache of the heart is a blessing that when accepted fully can be shared with all." Having a raw and open heart didn't feel very much like a blessing at first, but I began to get used to it. I slowly learned to trust that I could acknowledge and hold the painful feelings that arose in me and survive.

One rainy day during this period of inner confusion, I was browsing through a downtown bookstore looking for some words of inspiration, and I picked up the book *The Wisdom of Insecurity* by Alan Watts. His words began to help me sit with the wide-open and tender spaces I was feeling inside of me—what Thich Nhat Hanh called aimlessness. Reading Watts's description of why we are here, corrected my misunderstanding of the term aimlessness. I realized now that it didn't mean nothingness or meaninglessness:

> At once it becomes obvious why this universe exists, why conscious beings have been produced, why sensitive organs, why space, time, and change. The whole problem of justifying nature, of trying to make life mean something in terms of its future, disappears utterly. Obviously, it all exists for this moment. It is a dance, and when you are dancing you are not intent on getting somewhere. You go round and round, but not under the illusion that you are pursuing something, or fleeing from the jaws of hell…the meaning and purpose of dancing is the dance. Like music, also, it is filled in each moment of its course.[2]

These words calmed my fears. And while I pondered them, unsure about how I might step fully out of my depression and participate in the world, we witnessed the events of September 11, 2001. Watching the surreal footage of the sudden and tragic deaths of so many people, my own life and the lives of my loved ones seemed more precious than ever before. The dance wasn't going to last forever. If I didn't find a way to get out of my mind and off my ass, I would miss it entirely.

Seitan Gyro a la Olga's Kitchen *(vegan)*

Olga's gyro was my absolute favorite food for many years while growing up. I later enjoyed lamb gyro when visiting Greece, which was even tastier. To replace the meat, I found a recipe for a Seitan gyro in Jo Stepaniak's book *Vegan Vittles: Down-Home Cooking for Everyone.* I adapted it over the years to get closer and closer to my own memory of Olga's classic lamb gyro. This is a favorite of mine served with rice or pita.

INGREDIENTS:

    4 ounces seitan strips

    ½ cup water

    ¼ cup soy sauce

    ½ teaspoon powdered garlic

    1 teaspoon oregano

    whole wheat or white pita bread

TOPPINGS:

    red onion, chopped finely

    tomatoes, chopped finely

    plain vegan yogurt (e.g., Wildwood)

METHOD:

Drain the seitan strips, rinse, and pat dry.

Heat a large skillet over medium-high heat.

Place the seitan in the skillet and stir until browned on all sides.

Mix together the water, soy sauce, and oregano.

Once the seitan is brown, add the soy sauce mixture, turn heat to low, and cover.

Let simmer until all the liquid is absorbed, about 5 minutes.

Serve in pita pockets with the toppings you like.

Serves 4.

Homemade Almond Milk (vegan)

I make almond (or other nut) milk every few days because I think it's much tastier than store bought; it is fresh, frothy, and has no additives or preservatives. I use it in coffee, tea, in recipes and smoothies, or on granola and other dry cereals. My daughters love it and have learned how to make it.

The downside is that it will only keep 3 to 7 days in refrigerators (use quickly!) and the cultivation of almond trees uses up a lot of precious water, especially in California. So I started playing with making milk from whatever nuts are most conveniently available. I happened upon a huge bag of raw pumpkin seeds (pepitas) and to my great surprise, they worked great in this recipe. I added a dash of nutmeg and cinnamon to the final milk. Yum.

INGREDIENTS:

1 cup raw organic almonds, rinsed thoroughly, then soaked in fresh filtered water for 3 to 12 hours (or use pumpkin seeds, cashews, or experiment with other nuts)

3 cups fresh filtered water

4 fresh dates

cheesecloth or nut bag

METHOD:

Rinse the almonds after they have finished soaking.

Place almonds, water, and pitted dates into blender and blend on the high or "juice" speed for 1 to 2 minutes, or until smooth.

Strain the almond milk through cheesecloth or a "nut bag" (easily purchased online) squeezing until only dried almond paste remains in the bag.

Drink or use in smoothies immediately, or store in glass jar in the refrigerator.

Note: If you find yourself with no cheesecloth, it is possible to make almond milk without straining the liquid, but it will contain a residue with similar texture to coffee grinds.

Makes approximately 3 cups.

Retreat–Style Oatmeal *(vegan)*

I learned how versatile oatmeal was when attending mindfulness retreats. Now I eat it all the time, and whenever we have guests staying with us in the winter, I mix up a big pot of it and set out whatever toppings I have so they can personalize their own breakfast.

It's so easy to make and perfect to carry with you if you have to be out of the house early. I sometimes prepare this before going to our 6:30 a.m. Wednesday morning meditation group. It gets cold and stiff while I'm sitting (and so do I!) and I warm it up by mixing in a few tablespoons of very hot or boiling water.

You can add almost anything to oatmeal and it still tastes good. My favorite additions are below, but don't let me stop you from adding anything sweet, salty, or even hot (like spicy cinnamon). I always add some kind of nuts or nut butter because the protein keeps me from getting hungry before lunch. Fresh or dried fruit adds the sweet flavor. Mix and enjoy!

Oatmeal generally comes in three varieties—quick-cooking, regular, and steel cut. This recipe is for regular oats, but if you want denser oatmeal, you can use steel cut, which takes about 20 minutes to cook. Quick-cooking oats aren't really necessary since regular oats only take a few minutes to cook on the stove. Follow the recipe on the back of the box to prepare quick-cooking or steel-cut varieties. (Soaking the oats overnight can cut down on the time needed for cooking in the morning.)

INGREDIENTS:

⅓ cup (organic) regular cut oats (gluten-free oats are often available in whole foods markets)

⅔ cup liquid (water, or water mixed with homemade almond milk for creamier oats)

dash of salt

1 tablespoon unsalted peanut butter or almond butter

1 tablespoon your favorite nuts, chopped into small pieces

1 tablespoon raisins (or other dried fruits, chopped into small pieces)

METHOD:

If preparing in advance, allow the oats to soak in the liquid overnight.

Add the oats and liquid to a small saucepan.

Add the salt and partially cover. (Covering completely may cause the oatmeal to boil over.)

Bring to a boil.

Reduce heat and let simmer mostly covered for 3 to 4 minutes, or until all liquid has been absorbed.

Cover fully and let rest for 1 to 2 minutes.

Spoon into your bowl and add the remaining ingredients. Enjoy!

For a weekend breakfast or brunch, add a serving of vegan sausage, like Gimme Lean Sausage or Smart Sausages by Lightlife.

4.

FROG on a PLATE

Today is a new day. You will get out of it just what you put into it. If you have made mistakes, even serious mistakes, there is always another chance for you. And supposing you have tried and failed again and again, you may have a fresh start any moment you choose, for this thing that we call "failure" is not the falling down, but the staying down.

—MARY PICKFORD

It's just after our nightly family dinner, and I pick up a dinner plate. The kitchen is overflowing with dirty dishes, all four kids are tearing around the house yelling and whining and definitely not doing their homework, and my husband and I haven't had sex in weeks. He was late for dinner tonight, as always, and now we are yelling at each other from across the kitchen. I feel the anger boiling up inside of me. I don't want to be there, and I don't want to keep arguing. I don't want to force the kids into doing all the things they don't want to do tonight. I've been eating nonstop since I began preparing dinner, and now I'm full and furious at myself. I just want to go to bed. Before I know it, the plate has left my hand and is flying angrily toward Paul's chest before it crashes into the wall, spewing a million pieces into the open dishwasher. Why am I so angry?

NEITHER PAUL NOR I CAN REMEMBER specifically what we were fighting about that night. I remember thinking that it was all Paul's fault. He was to blame for all of my unhappiness. "If only he could come home on time. If only he could help me more with the kids. If only he could stop telling me what to do." It felt better to think that everything bad was his fault than that I was angry or depressed.

I worried about whether our family was okay. Paul's CPA father euphemistically called us "passionate," and we were definitely that. Lucile started rebelling at nine ("I don't give a damn what you say, I am not going to soccer practice!"), Jamie was developing a distressing perfectionism ("I'm *soooo stuuupid!*"), Veronica couldn't eat off plates that were white, and Louie was sent home from kindergarten for looking up girls' dresses. It was hard to resist thoughts of checking out when there were so many strong emotions.

Paul escaped to work, perfecting the traditional role of provider, which put me in the position of managing all the child-care and household responsibilities along with my graduate schoolwork. I loved my family, but I was lonely, tired, and annoyed. I thought my new mindfulness practice would make me feel better, but so far it had been more like taking the cork out of a bottle of champagne. My emotions still had to bubble over for a while before they could settle back down. With mindfulness, my feelings seemed so much more tangible than they had been when I was suppressing them with food and alcohol. Sometimes I could notice them and not act on them, but sometimes I couldn't help but react.

This was one of those times that I could see my emotion, my fury at my husband, and I was conscious that I was about to do something I'd have to apologize for later. I could feel it coming, but I didn't have enough mindfulness practice under my belt to be able to stop it. I saw the plate; I felt the anger. My spacious mind said, "This is anger," and my reptilian brain said, "Throw it at him!" I picked up the plate, my jaw tensed, and I felt a moment of power in my hands, just what I needed. I wanted to stop there, but the neural pathways of anger were too well worn, and I let the plate go. It was major progress that I was now aware of my feelings and my impulses to act on them—I just couldn't control the outcome yet.

This incident was a perfect example of the second arrow and the power of conditioning. My annoyance at the situation, my fatigue, and my loneliness were uncomfortable emotions. Instead of just taking care of my own feelings, I shot myself with the second arrow. I blamed my husband for all of it. I told myself that it was his fault. For a short time my anger felt really good, but the loneliness and fatigue didn't go away. They were simply compounded by the feelings of shame and isolation that arose after the plate came smashing down and Paul retreated. In time I was able to change those patterns, but it didn't happen overnight.

September 12

On September 11, 2001, I decided that if I was going to change my life, I had to do it now. Being in Washington, DC, on that day was terrifying. Paul and I had been on a day trip to Pennsylvania when the Pentagon was hit by a plane, and our kids, who had been released early from school to another family, were more than relieved to see us when we got home. Like a slap in the face, September 11 woke me up and propelled me into my true vocation. Although I was a relative beginner to mindfulness and yoga, I had seen mindfulness practitioners keep their calm in difficult situations and I passionately wanted more people, especially children, to know how to avoid conflicts like the ones that led to 9/11.

The only person I could think of who might help me get started was the peace activist and former *Washington Post* columnist Colman McCarthy, whom I had heard of, but had never met. Colman taught courses on alternatives to violence at several local colleges and public high schools. I found his email address online, and sent him a note asking how I could bring mindfulness, nonviolent communication, and yoga to young people in DC.

Colman connected me to a woman who was guiding the peer mediation programs in several DC public schools, and I began to assist her weekly groups. At the same time, I began a weekly program in Louie's second-grade class focused on teaching conflict resolution through mindfulness and non-violent communication.

During the months following 9/11, Washington, DC, experienced more frightening events, including deadly sniper and anthrax attacks, and I continued to bring what I was learning about mindfulness to the classroom. I expanded my teaching to provide programming for all the other second-grade classes, and later I started kid's yoga classes, one at the school and another at a nearby gym. Eventually I opened a mindful yoga studio for kids, families, and adults. I was always just one step ahead of my students, who inspired me to continue learning and practicing more so that I could pass what I learned along to them.

Meanwhile, I continued to bring my own children on mindfulness retreats, and I began attending a weekly meditation group. I also went to church now and then, though most of the time without Paul or the kids, who preferred to stay home on Sundays. I still wanted the familiarity of a Christian church, but meditation and mindfulness just made more sense to me. Eventually, I gave up church altogether.

Our family mindfulness practices began to truly take hold, especially around the dinner table. Each evening we paused to give thanks for our meal—saying either a familiar Christian grace ("Dear God, I'm glad you are always here. Help me to know and do the things that are right and good"), a song ("The Lord Is Good to Me"), or the Five Contemplations before Eating (see Appendices, page 236). Then one of us would ring a small meditation bell, marking the beginning of one minute we spent eating in silence. We called it "thinking time," though of course it was meant to be mindful eating time. Not everyone liked it. Lucile often rolled her eyes, but she kept quiet.

At the end of the minute, we again rang the bell, and after most of us had finished eating, each person shared about their day. They could tell us what they had done or they could sing their day in a made-up tune. Although we sat at the very same wooden table that I had grown up eating dinner on, we were creating a completely different kind of meal tradition—one that included mindfulness.

Angeles Arrien taught me a powerful ancestral song about changing family dynamics that has been an inspiration for me as I keep trying to alter our family patterns of compulsive eating, even if the changes are small:

Oh may this be the One who will bring forward
the good, true, and beautiful in our family lineage;
Oh, may this be the One who will break the harmful family patterns,
or harmful cultural patterns.
Oh, may this be the One.

Frogs

Thich Nhat Hanh offers insight into how the mind works in his poem "Froglessness" (see Appendices, page 237). When a frog is put on a plate, it naturally jumps off the plate. So we gently put the frog back on the plate. Again it jumps off. And again we put it back. This is exactly how we learn to keep our minds in the present moment. The practice is simply to return our minds to our focus—whether it's on a bite of oatmeal, our son's guitar solo, or our fear about being in the dentist's chair—without judging or condemning ourselves for having a wandering mind. It's the nature of the frog to jump. Likewise, it's the nature of our minds to wander.

In theory, mindfulness is simple. It's being awake for what is happening in this moment—what we are thinking, saying, feeling, experiencing, or doing. It is nonjudgmental awareness. We may not like what is happening, but instead of avoiding it, we simply notice that we don't like it. When we can be mindful in the kitchen, cooking or eating can become a form of meditation. When we cook, we are present with our cooking. When we eat, we are present with our eating. We let go of the habit of thinking, worrying, judging, and planning, and we simply experience the moment, regardless of whether we find it pleasant or unpleasant.

If your food tastes delicious, you enjoy it. If you overcook the kale and it tastes like rubber, you may not like it (or want to eat it), but you remain curious. "Hmm, burned kale tastes like this." This is how we practice staying with the first arrow, not allowing the second one to hit. I began to notice how I felt after compulsive eating: "This is what it feels like to be bloated." I experienced it directly. It wasn't a good feeling.

The fact is, many moments involve feelings that aren't particularly pleasant. But we don't have to react or shoot ourselves with the second arrow every time we have an unpleasant feeling. When we're mindful, every moment is an opportunity to learn about our experience and practice detachment—being with the feelings but not carried away by them.

Food is a great vehicle for mindfulness. But eating mindfully isn't easy, trust me. I've been practicing for almost twenty years, and only now and then do I do it well. The easiest way to start is by paying attention to our senses. Consider the taste of an apple. Now try to describe what it tastes like. It's not easy to describe. If you take a bite of an apple, however, you instantly know what an apple tastes like, right? Tasting happens in the body first, and then later our mind labels it an apple.

When you are eating that apple, just experience the apple, not your thoughts about the apple. If you notice that you're thinking about the stupid thing you said to your boss earlier, or the annoying way your daughter looked at you this morning, you are missing your one and only encounter with this apple. Why resist enjoying the apple fully? Why let your mind shift back into ruminating about what's wrong or right with your life when a delicious apple is right there in your mouth? When we simply taste the apple, we are aware of it in the present moment and we aren't thinking about the idea of an apple, or about anything else.

Eugene Gendlin, author of *Focusing*, calls this the "felt sense" of the moment. A felt sense is always more than words can describe. It includes everything we can experience: physical sensations, thoughts, and feelings. A felt sense is an inner knowing, or what he called, a "body-sense of meaning."[3] We have to be in the moment to experience the felt sense of it.

When I was bingeing, I could eat a dozen pancakes swimming in syrup in just a few bites. I might have experienced the first bite, but after that my mind was racing either to the future ("What will I eat next?") or the past ("Why didn't my boyfriend call me?") or lost in self-judgment ("I'm so fat/ stupid/gullible/ugly"). Most of my binge was spent ruminating in my mind just so I could avoid my feelings. The good news is we can relearn to eat and enjoy food.

I often teach a simple practice to kids called an "M&M Ceremony" in which we get the felt sense of eating a single M&M. We slow down the process and use all our senses to really take that M&M. It's the opposite of bingeing. We look at our M&M, we smell it, and finally we taste it. We let it linger in our mouth without chomping it down, and we savor whatever flavors arise. Whenever our mind drifts off to think about something else, we bring it back to the taste of the M&M, just like putting the frog back on the plate. (Directions for having a Mindful Chocolate Ceremony are on page 114). You can also use a raisin or a tangerine instead of a piece of chocolate here, depending on your or your kids' taste.

Mindfulness is the practice of staying with what is in the present moment, recognizing when our mind wanders, and coming back to the present moment again. We learn to recognize when we are tasting something, we recognize when we are thinking, and we learn how to bring our attention back to tasting again. Over time, our mind gets used to coming back and we can maintain attention on our food for longer periods of time.

When we are able to do this, we very often eat less and enjoy our food more. That's because we are eating only what our body really wants and needs. We are no longer mindlessly stuffing food in our mouths.

A student once asked me, "What if I like thinking about my work project while I'm eating an apple? Is there anything wrong with that?" I thought that was a great question. To me, mindfulness is all about choice. If you want to think about your work project, then think about your work project. But if you want to enjoy your apple but you can't because you are thinking about your work project, then mindfulness helps you bring your mind back to the apple.

If we manage to really experience this moment, to really taste the apple or the M&M, chances are we'll be more present to experience our next moment, whether it's an apple, a concert, or a good-night kiss from a loved one. As Thich Nhat Hanh says, "The best way to take care of the future is to take care of the present moment."

I have eaten thousands of meals during which I ate a lot but tasted nothing. I might have been worrying about how I could afford to buy groceries when we were behind on our mortgage or whether my son was mad at me for not letting him have another sleepover. Not only did I lose the chance to enjoy the food in front of me, but I didn't solve the problems I was worrying about. All I did was reinforce my habit of thinking instead of being present for my meals and my life. The wise eighth-century Buddhist teacher Shantideva said, "If the problem can be solved, why worry? If the problem cannot be solved, worrying will do you no good." When eating, just eat—don't worry. When the frog jumps off the plate, it's not a problem. Just put him back on it.

Lighten Up and Grieve

Once you start putting the frog back on the plate, you and the frog both begin to get trained. He still jumps, but a little less frenetically, and you trust that if he jumps, you will notice and will be able to put him back on the plate without any drama. With this new faith in your practice, you will be able to see life more clearly. The word "buddha" means awake. What the Buddha taught was how to be awake to our life. Most of us are sleeping through our lives—and we keep hitting the snooze button!

A young American Buddhist monk told me, "Once you see the true nature of your mind, you can't help but laugh." The absurd ways my mind tries to cope with life are truly laughable. But it's also true that once you see the true nature of your mind, you can't help but cry. Thich Nhat Hanh's poem, "Please Call Me by My True Names" highlights this paradoxical truth:

Please call me by my true names,
so I can hear all my cries and laughter at once,
so I can see
that my joy and tears are one.

As my mindfulness stabilized, I could see the humor in my life, and sometimes laugh about it. At other times I cried when I faced the pain I was carrying from my youth, the food dysfunction in our family, or the suffering of the millions of people and animals who are forced to bear truly awful situations. I learned how to live with both the pain and the laughter in my life by learning to sit still with whatever situation I encountered.

My dear friend Reverend Julia Jarvis says that fifty percent of life is grieving. That doesn't mean that we spend half of our lives depressed, but it does mean that we have to learn how to be with our own, and eventually with others', sorrows and unmet needs. Instead of chasing after what we don't have or can't get, or judging ourselves as lacking and making ourselves depressed, we fully accept and mourn the fact that we may not have all the life circumstances we thought we would. Whether it's having the squat body of our mother instead of the tall slim shape of our father, losing someone we love dearly, or not having the close relationship we thought we would have with our child, mourning what we can't change is how we begin to lessen the wound from the first arrow.

By taking time to mourn, we let go of trying to control the uncontrollable. Once we stop trying to force our life to be different than it is, we can tap into the wisdom that will help us take the next step. Marshall Rosenberg puts it this way: "The practice is to be able to empathize with ourselves and our needs that have not been met…to learn to mourn without self-blame."[4]

The Three Contemplations

There are three things that the Buddha wanted us to remember about life:

1. Sometimes life sucks (The insight of Dissatisfaction)
2. Nothing lasts (The insight of Impermanence)
3. We're all in this together (The insight of Interbeing or Interdependence)

Sometimes Life Sucks (The Insight of Dissatisfaction)

Although the wind blows terribly here, the moonlight also leaks between the roof planks of this ruined house.

—IZUMI SHIKIBU

In 2003 I took the kids to a retreat at the Plum Village monastery in rural southwest France. Plum Village is Thich Nhat Hanh's Zen community situated in the midst of vineyards and sunflower fields. The buildings are old, rustic, and charming, in the characteristic architecture of this region of France.

It was the hottest summer on record in Europe since 1590—literally thousands of people in France tragically died from the heat that year—and we were given a stifling room to share with another family. In total our room housed two adults and six kids between the ages of ten and thirteen. There was no air conditioning in any building, and our room had only one small window. The girls slept in bunk beds in the sweltering hot, windowless loft.

I was put into the work group that chopped vegetables outside the kitchen building in the evenings, when it was coolest. We chopped vegetables for two hours each evening on an old wooden table under the shade of a rickety tin roof. The cooks used our cut vegetables for the community's many delicious vegetarian dishes, including chickpea stew and tofu with mushrooms.

I loved the communal chopping of carrots, zucchini, and herbs, many of which were grown in the garden behind the kitchen. Before they were washed, the vegetables smelled of earth; and the rhythmic sound of chopping on wood was soothing. Breathing in, I chop; breathing out, I smile. We worked in silence, and I was able to connect with the food I was preparing beyond simply seeing its utility for the meal.

We were instructed to enjoy our breathing while we chopped, to work in silence, and to use concentration and care in how we cut each vegetable—but not to be perfectionistic about it. Being a perfectionist is just another distraction, another way of getting caught by our thinking, and comparing ourselves to an ideal standard instead of being in the present moment. Our little group of ten volunteers chopped vegetables and breathed together in the slightly cooler night air.

On the fourth evening of our retreat, one of the hottest, I was chopping vegetables with my team when Lucile found me to ask if she could spend the night in the woods with a bunch of other teenagers. When I said no, she went ballistic. Over the course of the next two hours, she screamed and swore at me. She slammed the door to our room repeatedly. I finished chopping and went to our room for Noble Silence—the period of time that begins after the evening activities and lasts through the following day's lunch, in which we enjoy silence. Lucile continued to make as much noise as she could. I felt anger and embarrassment rising in me. I wanted to grab her by the shirt and scream, "Shut the hell up!" in her face.

Sometimes things happen in life that are challenging. Sometimes it's blazing hot and you have to sleep in a loft without a window on the hottest night in four hundred years. And then your stupid mom won't let you sleep outside with all the other kids. Sometimes your daughter yells at you and keeps the whole silent retreat awake. Nothing that happens *to* us can be controlled. Sometimes good things happen and sometimes not-so-good things happen. This is what the Buddha wanted us to remember. Because only when we stop trying to control what comes at us can we put our energy where we can really make a difference: in our reaction.

Of course, terrible things happen too, like a tsunami or the death of someone we love. But for the most part we recognize that we have no control over life-changing events. It's really the small- and medium-sized challenges that hook us into thinking that if we just tried hard enough, we could prevent them. But we can't.

I didn't know where to turn, so I went back to the vegetable-chopping table and sat down. Some of the other choppers were still there, and we spoke a little, but mostly we just sat together in our makeshift "kitchen." After an hour of quiet, I felt much calmer, and I was able to speak calmly to Lucile about why I said no. Though I normally would have been very reactive in such a situation, I was able to hear her anger and not become rigid and controlling or escalate the situation by verbally firing back.

More than just being with the people in my group (though they were important), I found that really being present with the vegetables grounded me. The daily practice of mindful cooking gave me the peace to be able to relax in the midst of my daughter's storm that erupted during our stay at Plum Village. She quieted down and finally fell asleep that night, but her complaints about the heat and everything else continued. On our last day, she announced that she was never going to another retreat. And she never did. I was disappointed, but for once, I had no parenting guilt, because I hadn't reacted impulsively to her anger.

Every day during that retreat I savored my time with the chopping team, and I ate all my meals silently and mindfully. I thought I had become a mindful eating professional! At the end of the week, we packed our bags and left, reaching the Bordeaux airport in time to grab whatever sandwiches we could and eat them quickly before boarding the plane. When we got home, I desperately clung to the shreds of mindful cooking and eating that I had known on retreat, but with jet lag, four hungry kids, and a full schedule at the yoga studio, my own mindful cooking and eating and once again slid into the background. It was always two steps forward and one step back. But at least I continued to move forward.

Something in me also felt guilty for wanting to spend more time cooking and eating. I felt I wanted to take time to cook and eat slowly and consciously, but I also had a voice in my head telling me that cooking and eating were a waste of time, and that I should be helping the world in a more direct way, like through politics or social action. That part of me still exists but over time I have befriended it—its job is to help keep me from becoming complacent. It's possible to take my time cooking and eating, to savor my time in the kitchen, and also to take on bigger world issues. In fact, I know now that the mindful time I enjoy in the kitchen energizes me for the bigger issues.

My body is one of the things that I can't entirely control. I will never be tall, have an hourglass figure, a flat stomach, or wear a small bra size, no matter what I do. There are forces in our genetics and our environment that affect how and where we gain weight. Some of us probably have a genetic predisposition to food cravings and overeating. Once we know which things we can and can't change, we can relax, work on what we can, and accept the rest.

As a young mother I was dissatisfied with so many things—my husband's lack of support being one of the big ones. What I know now is that even if I had a husband who came home early or did all the laundry, I would have been dissatisfied with something else. Things are going to arise that push our buttons. We are hardwired for dissatisfaction. There is no way to avoid it.

I don't know all the factors that led to my bulimia and compulsive eating, but if I hadn't had an eating disorder, there would have been something else.

I remember in my class on grief and loss at Howard, we went around the room and each of us was asked to tell the class what "cross" we were bearing in this lifetime. Everyone had something. We all do.

There is no way to get rid of our cross, but there is a way to bear it more lightly. The first step is to recognize that we are much more than our burden. As I practiced mindfulness I became aware of the difference between the thoughts that caused me to suffer and the "real me" who watched the thoughts. It was only when I separated these two that "I" could turn toward the suffering part of myself with compassion and start to transform her. When we can take care of the wound from the first arrow, we won't shoot ourselves with the second arrow.

While my kids were growing up, I was either working or in graduate school. I got up early to meditate, went to class or worked, then ran errands or grocery shopped, and showed up at the kids' school in time for the 3:20 afternoon pick-up bell. Each day when we walked in the door together around 3:45, I realized I was exhausted. I had almost no energy in reserve for my kids, but they were all in desperate need of attention from Mommy and hours of chauffeuring were about to begin. To avoid focusing on my exhaustion and guilt (and my covert anger toward kids that I couldn't say no to), I made a beeline to the kitchen for a "snack." I sometimes still do this. When I got into the house, I was briefly released from my incessant work and to do list, and I felt anxious about what I should be doing next. Instead of sitting with the anxiety, I went for the food. Eating kept me in a state of distraction. Whenever there was a pause in activity, I'd head back to the kitchen for another little diversion.

This is a normal time of day to feel hunger and eat something, a low blood sugar time of day. But I wasn't usually hungry for food; I just didn't want to feel whatever was upsetting me. It could have been worry about one of the kids, an argument with my mom, or stress about money. When I was busy and working, I didn't have to pay attention. While cooking, I continued to numb myself with food, and by the time we had dinner, I wasn't hungry at all. Why would I be? I had eaten several meals before we sat down to eat.

To keep up the pretense of my "normal" relationship with food, I filled my plate and ate it anyway.

But gradually, as I continued to practice mindfulness and meditation, there began to be times when I could briefly stay with my difficult feelings. I found out that many of the feelings didn't last long if I gave them my full attention and compassion. Some only took a few minutes to soften. They didn't usually disappear, but by turning toward my feelings rather than turning toward the muffins, I began to figure out what I was really hungry for.

Thich Nhat Hanh describes this process as taking care of our baby. When we "pick up" our anxiety, fear, sadness, inadequacy, or other strong emotions the way we would pick up a crying baby—with tenderness and curiosity—it changes. Just like a baby responds to being picked up, our emotions respond to our mindful attention. Sometimes a baby just needs comfort, and sometimes our feelings just need to be heard and accepted. At other times, the baby needs something more, like a diaper change, and sometimes our feelings need more too—but we can only know this after we pick them up and offer some supportive, loving care.

The more I've practiced this skill, the less I have had to squash my strong emotions with food or other distractions. Practicing "picking up the baby" when we are triggered by strong emotions is very helpful. But, just like running a marathon, it's easier to do if we've had some training with lower-stakes emotions. Meditation is how we train ourselves to develop the skill of being with strong emotions. Meditation builds our mindfulness muscle in the same way that doing consistent, short training runs prepares us for a longer run.

Your cross to bear, your suffering, may look different from mine, but that's just its disguise. We all want to avoid feeling pain and to live in peace. It's only when we learn to be comfortable with the awkwardness and complexity of life and stop tiptoeing around every feeling are we able to fully live. Hidden just behind our tender hearts is a vast expanse of contentment, waiting for us to find it.

Nothing Lasts (The Insight of Impermanence)

Ah the knowledge of impermanence that
haunts our days is their very fragrance.

—RILKE

The second contemplation recommended by the Buddha is on the imper-manence of life: Everything we can see and know is subject to change; noth-ing stays as it is forever.

One winter, when the kids were still in elementary school, we took a family ski trip to Vermont. On the day we were scheduled to leave, our return flight to DC was canceled because of a terrible snowstorm. Rather than stay overnight and wait for the next flight, we felt we needed to get home, so we decided to rent a minivan and drive more than five hundred miles in a blizzard.

Everyone had fallen asleep as I cruised along, driving much faster than I should have been, on the deserted, snowy highway coming out of the moun-tains. I could see only a few feet in front of the car because of the dark night and the densely swirling snow. Suddenly, I hit a patch of ice and lost control of the car. Our van was spinning back and forth across the highway. It was a "Jesus, Take the Wheel" moment.

For the next several seconds, which felt like hours, we rebounded between the piles of snow that padded the guardrail and the ones along the shoulder. I thought to myself, "What a shame that our family is going to die here on the New York Interstate." Then I silently chastised myself: "I should have been driving slower." And then I experienced a bittersweet sadness—I was already grieving the loss of our amazing family and each of our lives. My sadness was mixed with gratitude for the love we all had for each other. Meanwhile, because I was raised in Michigan and was therefore familiar with driving in dangerous conditions, the unconscious part of my brain was instructing my hands in how to keep the car from flipping. Somehow, I found the highway under my wheels again. I had regained control of the car.

Paul and all four kids woke up during the spinning. When I felt the road again, I whispered to Paul that I was back in control of the van. Everyone stayed eerily silent. The release of fear cause me to be overcome with nausea and I felt like I would throw up, but it passed and we continued to drive on through the darkness. No one said a word, and no one fell back asleep. We had sat on the razor's edge between life and death. I believe each one of us knew that our survival had been in question that night. Two hours of silent gratitude passed before anyone spoke. We crossed into Pennsylvania and Veronica shouted, "We in Penny!" The spell was broken, and what remained was a visceral realization of the fragility of this life. For once, I really knew in my gut that it would all be over some day. Luckily, that wasn't the day, and we arrived safely home in DC.

When I was newly married and my mother was still alive, my husband and I went back to Michigan for Thanksgiving, to my maternal grand-mother's house on the St. Claire River in the picturesque small town of Algonac, where I had spent every Thanksgiving of my life up to that point. My grandparents' white clapboard house looked across the street toward the river where my grandpa's gas station and tackle shop had operated for decades.

My grandpa died when I was about ten years old, and I didn't know my dad's parents, so the only grandparent I ever really knew was my grandma. She looked a lot like a picture-book grandma—short and soft, usually wear-ing an apron and beehive white hair. She always had a warm, open smile when her grandkids showed up. I loved my grandma more than anyone else, and I felt she knew me better and loved me more than my own parents did.

From the time I was very young, my parents worked hard and were often distracted by their jobs and activities, so they didn't know a lot about my life. My grandma, on the other hand, though she had eighteen grand-children, called and wrote me regularly and asked about my friends by name. Twenty-five years after her death, I still know her phone number by heart. She sewed each of her grandchildren a piece of clothing or a robe for Christmas, and she cooked and baked delicious meals for every holiday, but absolutely the very best gifts were her hugs. Upon arriving and leaving

Grandma's house, we each enjoyed the plushest, most loving Grandma bear-hug embrace you can imagine. Neither of my parents was very physical, so for me this hug was like water to a parched woman in the desert.

Her old house was always warm and welcoming. You entered the side door, directly into her large country kitchen. To the left you could see into her living room and out the window to the river. To the right was her kitchen, her pantry, and the unheated "back room," which was freezing nine months of the year. This was where she stored her root vegetables in the winter and where we cousins ate Thanksgiving dinner. The door to her one bathroom, complete with clawfoot tub, was right beside her stove. Just before you reached the back room were stairs to the large unfinished basement, which housed a smallish room lined with wooden shelves that were always full of preserved food. She canned everything—tomatoes, rhubarb, berries, pickles—but sadly I never learned this art from her.

I didn't know it then, but this visit with my new husband was the last Thanksgiving I would ever spend with Grandma. In fact, I didn't see my grandma alive again. As usual, she cooked and baked most of the delicious food for the meal. My mom brought her special baked onions and cheesy cabbage, and my aunt Debbie brought her usual tiny plate of brownies. Of course, Grandma made the pies.

My favorite of her pies was pumpkin. It was smooth, unpretentious, and not too sweet. You could really taste the pumpkin, and most of the pie's sweetness came from the hand-whipped cream we liberally spooned on top. Only a handful of my twenty cousins joined us that last year, so everyone sat at the "adult" table. I ate my meal and my pie and hung out at the table chatting with my family. I know the pie must have been good, because it always was, but I'm not sure how much of it I really tasted.

Had I known that I was eating a piece of the last pumpkin pie my grandma would ever make, I would have savored the hell out of that pie. I would have given my full attention to the pie while I ate it, rather than devouring it while talking. I would have eaten it slowly and mindfully, memorizing the taste. Had I known it was my last piece, I would have enjoyed it more.

But what I would have savored most of all were my grandma's love-packed hugs. I missed her hugs so much after she was gone that one night, not long after she passed away, I dreamed that I was at her house. It was late, and my grandma knew that she was going to die, but she wanted to give me one last hug. She held me close to her, just as she always had. I breathed in a combination of perfume powder and baked chicken. We let go and she returned to her bedroom to lie down and die. I woke up feeling grateful, as though I'd enjoyed a bonus hug from Grandma (see page 208 for Hugging Meditation).

This is what the Buddha wanted us to remember about impermanence. Nothing lasts. We know this, but we forget and then we act as though nothing is changing. Kay Ryan's poem "The Niagara River" describes this delusion in a metaphor: we are floating along a river, not paying attention to the fact that we are headed straight for Niagara Falls.

... We
do know, we do
know this is the
Niagara River, but
it is hard to remember
what that means.

The fact is, we never know if we'll get to hug our beloved again or eat another piece of Grandma's pie. We don't know whether this is the last meal that we'll ever cook for our ourselves or our loved ones. All we know is that in this moment we have something precious, whether it's a deeply delicious slice of lovingly baked pie or someone at our kitchen table who loves us enough to eat our slightly burned pancakes, as my family did for decades.

Our feelings are impermanent too. This is good news, especially when I am so angry I want to throw my phone in the toilet or so sad I can't get out of bed. It's nice to remember that my uncomfortable feelings won't last forever—but pleasant feelings like joy, playfulness, and excitement are also impermanent. When I remember how transient all my feelings are, I'm not as likely to gauge my life by them. I can be content when I'm feeling sad and when I'm feeling joyful. When we know that nothing lasts, we don't bother pushing away what we don't like or clinging to what we like. We let it all roll by on the way to Niagara Falls.

When my mother was dying at a hospital in Florida, my sisters and I gathered there with my father. We knew her prognosis was very bad, and we decided to have some coffee in the hospital cafeteria while we waited for her cardiac test results. Although we had been scared and sad for the last twenty-four hours, when we got the call to come upstairs to say our final good-byes, we were in the midst of laughing about how our mother used to pack our refrigerators with low-fat food whenever she visited. Even in such a dismal situation, our emotional states were not permanent or fixed. We can be laughing one minute and sobbing the next. As the adage goes, and as my mom always said, "This too shall pass."

Each time I look in a mirror, I'm reminded of impermanence. I see new wrinkles, more back and upper belly fat, less butt, and more age spots (oh yay!). Medical science estimates that cells in our body die and regenerate such that we have an entirely new body every seven years. For example, although my skin cells are defined by my DNA and passed down to me from my parents, the actual matter of my skin is created by what I eat, whom I touch, and the dust and debris that falls on me.

The kitchen is a great place to see impermanence at work: the herb seeds I planted last year, to my surprise and delight, have become an herb garden. The kale in my refrigerator turns yellow and rank when I don't eat it soon enough. When I throw the kale into the compost, it becomes dense nutritious compost that would have been wonderful food for my new plants if I hadn't missed the window of time for planting!

When we eat, our food breaks down and becomes part of us. Our digestive tract absorbs nutrients, sending signals to our brains about hunger and fullness (often too late to prevent us from finishing the coconut ice cream). The feeling of fullness activates neurotransmitters in our brain that trigger feelings based on our conditioning. If our minds have the habit of feeling happy when we're full, then we feel happy. If our neurotransmitters are in the habit of creating a feeling of unhappiness when we're full, we'll feel unhappy. After eating, we might start sweating or emitting smells as our food breaks down. Nothing is destroyed during this process, just transformed. Every part of the meal is used somewhere!

Nourishing ourselves with food is the ultimate impermanent task. We are full one moment and hungry again the next. We make breakfast and before we know it, it's time to make lunch. Then it's dinnertime. Impermanence is woven into the fabric of life. Change is the only definite. We can bemoan this reality, or we can embrace the possibilities of change, savoring every moment.

Impermanence also makes it easier to accept our limitations and imperfections, because no mistake defines us forever. As the mystic poet Rumi said: "Ours is not a caravan of despair. Come, even if you have broken your vows a thousand times. Come, yet again, come, come." Because of impermanence we can be, and truly are, reborn in each moment.

We're All In This Together (The Insight of Interbeing or Interdependence)

> *It really boils down to this: that all life is interrelated.*
> *We are all caught in an inescapable network of mutuality,*
> *tied together into a single garment of destiny. Whatever*
> *affects one directly, affects all indirectly. We are made*
> *to live together because of the interrelated structure*
> *of reality…Before you finish eating breakfast in the*
> *morning, you've depended on more than half the world.*
>
> —MARTIN LUTHER KING, JR.

If nothing lasts, who and what are we? Our physical bodies, our thoughts, and our emotions are constantly in flux. Even our most stable personality traits, like my love of reading or my introversion, were passed down from previous generations or are habits we develop during this lifetime. There is really nothing permanent or fixed or inherent to me that I can label as "Annie" except a process of ever-changing physical matter, feelings, and thoughts that interact with and are modified by other matter, feelings, and thoughts.

This is the third contemplation given by the Buddha: We're all intimately connected because none of us is a separately divisible entity. Everyone and everything is dependent on everything else. Although we live in a very independent-minded culture, the truth is that we're actually like newborn babies, unable to do anything by ourselves.

Let's say you're eating some of those M&M's from the M&M Ceremony right now. You bought them with money that you made at your job, and you walked to the store to buy them. It seems like you did this all by yourself. However, if you look a little more closely, you will see that the entire universe had a hand in this moment of crunching a little blue candy.

To start with, your parents obviously had a part. Without them and their DNA, you wouldn't be here at all—the same is true for all your ancestors all the way back to the beginning of time. Without your parent's love, and frankly, without their sexual desire, you would never have been created. To love each other as they did, they had to have known some role models, so whoever your parent's role models were, they are in this moment of M&M eating too. And that's just for starters. You could take this in infinite directions going back in time forever.

What about the M&M's? Some factory workers had their hands literally on these very M&M's at the Mars candy factory. Forrest Mars himself, along with his ancestors, are here with you too. Without their creativity and money, this bag of M&M's would never have been possible. And if M&M's never existed, neither would this particular version of you. Do you follow? The chocolate manufacturer, the cacao tree growers, the people who pick the cocoa beans, the people who invented chocolate, many other people, and the trees themselves, are part of this moment.

Someone in your past must have introduced you to M&M's, or you wouldn't know how good they are. Don't forget the person who hired you at your job, and the one who wrote the check, and the bank who cashed the check, and the teller who gave you the cash (or the person who developed the ATM and built it, etc.) that allowed you to buy the M&M's. All those people are here too.

Your ability to digest the M&M's is dependent on the food you ate in the past, the people who grew and cooked it, the plants and animals who gave their lives and the more than one hundred trillion microbes living in, on, and around you, and the health of your microbes affects your ability to enjoy these M&M's. I am even there with you in this moment because you are reading this book and ingesting my words.

This is often the most difficult contemplation for us to fully and completely understand. We usually feel like we are separate from other beings, and in one sense we are. My body is over here and yours is over there. We aren't the same person. In another sense, however, we can't be separated from all the other people, plants, and places that make us who we are in each moment. Both are true: We are separate people, and we are dependent on everything and everyone else to continue to exist.

What we cook and eat is not separate from us either. How we cook and what we eat can make us healthy or unhealthy, happy or sad, alert or fatigued. And what we eat can make a difference in our lives and the world at large. Mindfully nourishing others contributes to our own happiness, as well as to a healthier world.

Our kids were baptized at a church that served weekly meals to the homeless community. For more than a decade our growing family cooked and served the weekly meal once a month on a Sunday afternoon. We prepared huge batches of chili or pasta for about eighty guests, and the kids helped us serve it from the church's back door. We all learned a lot about interdependence on those Sundays.

One winter day, a man came in wearing shoes with no soles. He asked if we knew anyone who was giving away shoes. Louie, then ten years old and already very fashion-conscious, was wearing his favorite pair of Timberland boots. When he saw how the man's socks touched the frozen ground, he took his boots off and handed them over. I was amazed because I am sure I would not have done the same thing at that age.

After serving, the men were invited into the church's dining room, and our kids often sat down to chat with them. There were at least two regular diners who were vegetarians, which surprised us. A kind older man named D.J. always brought the kids little trinkets he found on the street—pens, clips, and other small items. By engaging these homeless men (and a few women) week after week, the children began to see that they weren't completely different from us. Now and then we would see one of the men out on the street in DC, and rather than being fearful, as they might have been otherwise, the kids began wanting to help. Once, when she was in seventh grade, Lucile came home, packed up two sack lunches, and ran to the local library to deliver them to a homeless man sitting outside.

Recognizing that we are all in this together can inspire our compassion and encourage us to reach out to those who need help. When we help someone else, we are helping ourselves. And when we help ourselves, we are helping others too.

Why Meditate?

When my son Louie was eleven, we were invited to join Thich Nhat Hanh on his first teaching tour to Vietnam in 2005 after forty years in exile from his country. Thay (meaning "teacher"), as he is known by his hundreds of thousands of students, was a monk in Vietnam during the French and American wars in Indochina. He campaigned globally for peace and was nominated for the Nobel Peace Prize in 1967 by Martin Luther King, Jr. In the 1960s, while he was speaking and teaching in the US, the Vietnamese government decided that Thay could not return home because he refused to take sides in the conflict. He eventually settled in southwest France, where he created the Buddhist monastery and retreat center of Plum Village. In the decades since its founding, he has continued to teach mindfulness, both in Plum Village and in countries around the world.

Along with the hundreds of monks and nuns from Plum Village, several dozen laypeople were invited to go on this trip. We couldn't afford to bring the whole family, and only Louie really wanted to go, so it was just the two of us. No one in our family had ever been to Southeast Asia, and Louie had been only as far as France.

On the flight over, I started feeling sick. After a fifteen-hour flight to Korea and a three-hour layover, we boarded another five-hour flight to Hanoi. Someone from the local mindfulness community picked the two of us up at the airport, and we squeezed with our bags into the back of what looked like a covered motorcycle. Naturally, it was raining.

By the time we wended our way through the crowded streets to our hotel, we were twelve time zones away from our home and I had a burning fever. Hanoi was much colder and damper than I had expected, and for some reason our hotel room was unheated. I couldn't find a thermostat any-where, and I was too exhausted to try to find someone who spoke English to ask, so we fell asleep shivering under our thin blankets.

That night, as my fever spiked, Louie and I both barely slept. We tossed and turned, waking every hour from the cold and jet lag. During one wake-ful period we thought we heard a ghost laughing. A few hours later it was time to get up.

It was Thich Nhat Hanh's first visit back to Vietnam since he had been exiled, and the government was monitoring our traveling community of mindfulness practitioners, so we were very rarely allowed to leave the group. We woke each morning at 5:00 a.m., in time to meet the buses taking us to the first temple where Thay would be teaching. His talks were in Vietnamese, of course, but we were given headsets for translation whenever possible. All of our meals were vegan and were prepared by local women from the temple. The dishes were cooked in giant pots over burners placed on the ground.

On this first morning, it was clear that I had the flu. I was bone-tired, feverish, and freezing, and Louie had serious jet lag. We were both very hun-gry since we hadn't eaten for at least twenty hours. We found our way down to the lobby in the dark, ready for our first 6:00 a.m. bus, which would take us somewhere, though we had no idea where. I was sick and anxious about being in such a strange and distant country, with no friends and no language skills and with only one of my kids. I can only imagine what it was like for

Louie, an eleven-year-old boy, seven thousand miles away from his home, his family and friends, and his video games.

There was no one in the lobby except the front desk clerk, who luckily spoke a little English. I asked about breakfast, and she brought us each a bowl of a green vegetable gelatin. When I looked at it, I felt nauseous. Louie was braver than I was, and possibly hungrier, and dove right in for a bite. I could see the look of surprise on his face, so I asked him, "What does it taste like?" Given our exhaustion, I expected him to spit it out, make a face, and demand some American cereal. But with a grin on his face, he replied, "It tastes like grass!"

This was a moment of mindful eating. Rather than adding a second arrow of blame, resentment, or anger, Louie simply tasted the food. He didn't lie and say he liked it. He just tasted it. He didn't weave some big dramatic story or call it "disgusting gelatinous crap." He stayed attentive and curious, and even found something funny about it. "This is what grassy gelatin tastes like." Cultivating the ability to stay stable and curious even during challenging situations is exactly why we practice meditation.

Practicing Sitting Still

To begin learning to sit still in meditation, we choose the easiest situation in which to be present. Dragging four kids through a mall, for example, isn't the easiest moment to practice. The easiest place to practice meditation is when and where we have the fewest external distractions. Being mindful in a quiet, peaceful space is easier than being mindful when we're already triggered. So that's how we start.

Zen meditation is generally done sitting cross-legged on a cushion, kneeling and using a meditation bench, or kneeling while straddling a cushion, and usually we face a wall or an altar (see Basic Sitting Meditation Practice, page 112). But you can start anywhere. I had a quiet living room with a comfy couch, so I started meditating there. After some months, I put a folded blanket on the floor of my bedroom in front of my grandma's old red bench. I had no idea what to put on the bench that wouldn't be distracting. Eventually I added a picture of my meditation teacher and a small statue of a peaceful-looking Buddha.

These days I have lots of other things on my meditation altar, including some mala beads brought back by Jamie from a Buddhist monastery in India, pictures of various other teachers who inspire me, a vase of something cut from my yard, and two round female figures. If you decide to make an altar, what you put there doesn't really matter as long as it adds to your mindfulness and ease and doesn't distract from your meditation.

Once you have cleared away as many external distractions as possible, try sitting down and see what happens. Most days, when I try to meditate, my mind is all over the place, and five minutes go by before I even realize I'm meditating. "Oh right, I'm supposed to be meditating here, not planning my day."

Sometimes I focus on the sounds around me to help me get into the present moment. Or I notice the warmth of my two little dogs curled up against me. My dogs help me sit every morning, because they are part of my routine. Each morning, we get out of bed, I brush my teeth, and then the three of us pad down the hall to my sitting area. When it's cold, I turn on the space heater and they have a blanket to lie on right next to where I sit. When the bell rings at the end of our sitting, they get up and we do some yoga stretches together. They always do upward dog and downward dog after our sitting. Then we go out for our morning walk.

At some point during my meditation I am able to bring my attention to my breathing. Breathing in, I feel I am breathing in. Breathing out, I feel I am breathing out. I do that until I notice I'm not with my breath anymore and instead I'm wondering whether I gave the dogs their flea medication this month. I smile, thinking that I'm just like everyone else with a mind that wanders, and then I bring my mind back to my breathing. I try not to berate myself for thinking about the fleas, the dogs, my kids, my parenting, my job, my parenting, the weather, my husband, my parenting yet again, or anything else. I just notice. Pretty soon the bell rings (I use a timer) and I get up and go about my day. After sitting meditation, I am more in touch with my steps as I walk from place to place, with whatever I am doing, and with my life. I have more awareness of what's happening in my mind, and why.

Sore Toes and More Second Arrows

By practicing meditation I can see more clearly what causes me to be reactive, and I can choose not to shoot myself with the second arrow. Everyone has different triggers. Dr. Sam, our family therapist, calls our triggers our "sore toes." They are the unique spots in us that are highly sensitive. When someone steps on our sore toe, it makes us want to shoot the second arrow— we might strike out, go on a binge, or blame ourselves.

Getting to know our sore toes helps us in several ways. We can find ways to take care of our sensitivities, like reaching out to a friend when we feel lonely. We can tell our loved ones which toes are sore, and how to avoid them. We can just have more compassion for our painful parts. Knowing our sore toes also helps us notice when they get stepped on, so that rather than shooting ourselves with the second arrow, we can acknowledge the pain and then tend to our sensitive areas.

Once, during a heated discussion, Paul stepped on my sore toe. He wasn't able to listen to what I was saying, even after I had said it thirteen times, and I suddenly felt a rush of anger and the desire to knock him off of his chair. But for the first time, because of my meditation practice, I sustained a moment of clarity. I felt my sore toe; and instead of grabbing Paul, I grabbed my standard poodle and ran out the door. I was furious as I walked with Gus around the block, but as I put a foot on each sidewalk square I brought my mind back to feeling my steps and my breathing. I said to myself, "This is what anger feels like," and "You poor thing, he stepped on your sore toe!" and I noticed how bad it felt in my body to be so angry.

As I walked, I didn't think about the details of the fight or who was right and wrong (though I was sure I was right), and I didn't even try to prepare my argument. I especially didn't keep saying to myself what an awful person Paul was for not understanding me, as I normally did. I only felt my steps and embraced my feelings with a lot of compassion. It took me at least twenty minutes to get around one block because I was walking so slowly.

When I got back to the house, I was a different person. I didn't need him to admit I was right or even listen to my side right then. I could be present and see that Paul was doing his best. My ability to be present diffused the anger bomb, and we found a way for both of us to get our needs met. Had I not taken that mindful walk, I am positive our fight would have escalated into something much uglier and created a longer-lasting schism between us. After this watershed moment, I found I was able to tend to my sore toes much more often. I can usually, but not always, recognize I am being triggered before I say or do anything at all, and remind myself that we are all doing our best. I sometimes wonder if I would still be married if I hadn't started practicing mindfulness.

This practice also changed my relationship to food, as eating is one of the main ways I act out when my sore toes get stepped on. Now, when I feel that soreness, I can take a break and say hello to my pain instead of just rushing to the cupboard for a big scoop of peanut butter. Having a sore toe hurts. When we first stop numbing ourselves with our addiction and start taking care of our sore toes instead, it's going to feel a little awkward, even uncomfortable. Developing the capacity to be comfortable with our discomfort takes patience and practice. It's what is sometimes called "the art of suffering."

Food is my outlet of choice, but it's certainly not the only way we might try to escape from discomfort. Anything can become an escape from our feelings—alcohol, drugs, sex, work, shopping, blaming, thinking and planning, reading, electronics, or surfing the Internet. We may use more than one way. When used as distractions, all of these become second arrows that cause more pain for everyone in the long run.

I saw my daughter shoot herself with a second arrow when her own bulimic behaviors surfaced. Lucile went to Ireland for a three-month stint as a nanny to four young kids. She was only eighteen, had never lived away from home before, and was lonely—the job was taxing for her. She was supposed to manage four kids, ranging from four years old to an oldest child, who was only a few years younger than Lucile. She had to cook and clean up after the whole family, take the little ones to school, and make sure the older ones got to all of their after-school activities.

Lucile didn't know how to hold her loneliness or handle the challenges of the job, and so she binged. Every time the family left her at the house, she ate. She tried to will herself to stop eating, but it wasn't her conscious mind deciding to eat. By the time she came home, she had gained more than thirty pounds and was seriously depressed.

Paul and I offered her a few options when she got home. She could go back to college, she could stay home and get a job, or she could go into treatment. To her great credit, she chose to go into treatment. It wasn't an easy choice for her or for the rest of our family, but it was there that she was able to learn how to sit still with her feelings, speak her truth, and treat herself more gently.

Now she is aware of when a binge is at hand or even in process, and she can compassionately take of herself. When she does eat compulsively, she knows that beating herself up will only make another episode more likely, so she simply lets that one go and gives herself a pass. Once she learned to recognize and take care of her sore toes, rather than distract herself from them by bingeing, she quickly lost the extra weight, and continues to be much happier with herself and more comfortable around food.

There's nothing inherently wrong with eating a pile of pancakes or a giant bowl of oatmeal, if you're truly hungry. But eating huge quantities of food out of avoidance or fear creates more unhappiness than it relieves. Setting mindful intentions helps by reminding us why we want to stay with a difficult emotion. We all have the habit of running away from difficult feelings—it's normal! But there is a huge payoff for learning to stay with them: We suddenly have the freedom to choose how to behave rather than following our usual unhealthy habits.

If the idea of eating an entire pizza or a loaf of bread pops into your head, instead of pushing it away ("Absolutely not, you loser!"), try turning toward the part of you that wants to eat, and say to yourself, "Oh sweetie, it sounds like you want to eat a lot right now. What do you really need?" Try opening up a dialogue with your sore toe. You may be surprised by what it has to tell you.

We also don't have to put so much importance on each feeling that arises. When you burn the chard, you simply burned the chard. When you are disappointed, you are simply disappointed. When you are lonely, you are simply lonely. There's nothing more to add. Our sore toes just crave our attention. Some sore toes may require support from friends, family, or counselors, and the ones that have been there longer may need more time to transform; but change begins by just giving them your undivided presence and attention.

You can't tell from looking at someone what sore toes they might have or what kind of second arrow they might be using to cover it up. People who looked at me or my daughters wouldn't have known that food was causing us so much suffering. In her book *Ravenous*, Dayna Macy reminds us, "It is a revelation to me that a 120-pound person and a 300-pound person can be similarly sad about their bodies. The thinner person may look like her act is more together, but pain is pain. Regardless of the number on the scale, few of us are truly happy and at home in the skin we're in." Meditation helps us get happier in our own skin and shoot ourselves with second arrows less often.

Setting Intentions

As you begin to practice meditation based on the Buddha's Three Contemplations—the insights of dissatisfaction, impermanence, and interdependence—you will notice old habits start to change. Understanding that life will always have challenges, that everything in the world is subject to change, and that we are dependent on the entire cosmos makes us more willing to stay with our difficult moments in order to be sure we don't waste our precious time. It's very easy to forget to practice the Three Contemplations—just as it can be hard to remember to practice mindfulness or to set aside time for meditation. We have to find a way to keep the Three Contemplations fresh in our lives.

Each morning, I open my journal and write my intentions for the day. Whether I'm cooking, teaching, or writing that day, it always helps to know what my intentions are. The first intention is usually something like, "Be as present as I can be today," or more specifically, "Pay attention to each step as I walk the dogs" or "Be present for my kids when they are talking to me." Intentions are the means by which we reach an end, but they are also an end in themselves. I forget my intentions many times during the day (heck, I'm glad if I remember them once), but setting them is more likely to keep them freshly in my awareness, and just having set them helps make a difference in how I go about my day.

A quick way that I remind myself of my intentions is by plastering sticky notes all around the house and car with reminders like, "This is it!" "Remember to breathe," "This cup of tea contains the entire cosmos," and "How important is it?"

Without intentions for our practice, we won't get very far. Our intentions direct our actions. The way we relate to each moment adds up to the way we live our lives. Taking one bite of food in mindfulness leads to another bite in mindfulness, which leads to eating an entire meal in mindfulness. Eating one meal in mindfulness leads to the next, and so on. How we relate to this moment, this bite, this recipe, and this emotion arising around food will determine how we feel about our eating and therefore our lives.

When my eating disorder was at its most profound, I didn't want to take even one bite in mindfulness because it meant that I would have to be aware of my body and all the negative stories circulating in my mind around eating and food. I was afraid that I wouldn't know how to be with those thoughts and feelings. By taking a conscious breath before I eat, I have learned how to be with my sore toes. I can stand to be present for my food more often because it's not just the food that I am being present for, but all the anxiety and self-judgment, the inner moaning and groaning, that's always spinning around in my mind.

Ten Thousand Hours of Pancakes

Once our kids were a certain age, they had sleepovers nearly every weekend. For a while we kept a six-person tent set up in our family room for just this purpose. At 2:00 a.m. one night, I decided to stop screaming, "Shut up and go to sleep!" (since it wasn't working), and instead I dragged myself downstairs and sang lullabies to them until they were lying still with their eyes closed. "See," I told myself, "you can catch more flies with honey than vinegar." Dropping onto my soft pillow, my eyes closed to the sound of Veronica's friend Ruth whispering to the other girls, "Get up, hey, get up." Within minutes all eight of them were back to full volume, and I went back to useless shrieking.

So most weekend mornings, I faced a crowd of hungry soccer players or sleepy teenagers. I found that pretty much everyone liked pancakes, so that became my go-to breakfast food on Saturday, Sunday, and summertime mornings. They were always a hit and very easy to make from scratch.

During the busiest years, I probably made a thousand pancakes a year. The most popular with the young kids, and even some adults, were the chocolate chip pancakes. Blueberry is now my son's favorite, though my husband only eats plain. (My son has even taught his French girlfriend—whom he met years ago at Plum Village—how to make them.) I can now mindfully whip up a batch of pancakes from scratch—dairy- and egg-free, gluten-free, or classic—in about a minute! It takes some time for the griddle to heat up, which is good because it gives me time to practice mindful breathing, get out the maple syrup, and set the table.

Mindfulness, like most disciplines and rituals, benefits from repetition. In his book *Outliers: The Story of Success*, author Malcolm Gladwell suggests that it takes ten thousand hours of practice to master any activity. I'm not sure I've reached ten thousand hours of pancake-making, but I'm getting close.

After practicing mindfulness for a few years, both on the cushion and at the griddle, it got easier to stay present. I started noticing how much more I was able to truly hear my children, even when they were angry at me. And, sure, I felt terrible about being told the truth—that I was ignoring them in favor of my computer or that I grilled their friends with too many questions. But I also felt something else: an authentic connection to people I loved.

Only when we are present can we experience the moment as it is. Learning how to train our attention isn't all that difficult, but it starts with noticing any time we aren't present. Once we notice we aren't present, then we can choose to bring our attention back again and again to whatever is happening, whether it's making a pancake, recovering from a grievance, or experiencing a hug.

In Charles Duhigg's book, *The Power of Habit*, he explains that it only takes doing something differently one time to change our conditioning. He quotes the famous behavioral psychologist and habit-reversal expert Nathan Azrin as saying, "It seems ridiculously simple, but once you're aware of how your habit works, once you recognize the cues and rewards, you're halfway to changing it. It seems like it should be more complex. The truth is, the brain can be reprogrammed. You just have to be deliberate about it." Mindfulness is the ability to become aware of and be deliberate about your habits.

Every time you do something differently you are literally changing your brain. In *Buddha's* Brain, Rick Hanson describes how mindfulness does this. "Mindfulness leads to new learning—since attention shapes neural circuits—and draws upon past learning to develop a steadier and more concentrated awareness. Wisdom is a matter of making choices, such as letting go of lesser pleasures for the sake of greater ones." Every time we put the frog back on the plate, we have a moment of wisdom in which we can make a new choice and strengthen the habit of making healthier and happier choices.

Into the Kitchen

I come to my kitchen the same way I come to my meditation cushion—accepting myself where I am. Sometimes I come into the kitchen angry at my husband, like the times he calls me just before dinner to say he is going to be an hour or two late, pushing everyone's bedtime and my "me time" to a later time. Sometimes I'm anxious about the future of the world because of the small and large injustices I see just about everywhere.

Sometimes I come into the kitchen exhausted because I had a particularly busy or stressful day, like my mom often did. Sometimes I come into the kitchen grieving the fresh loss of one of our parents or a beloved dog. In each case, I still do the same things—determine what the menu for the meal will be, collect the ingredients, prepare the meal, and eat it. My feelings may remain there in the background, held with my self-compassion, but I try to keep the food itself—its taste, smell, texture, and colors—in the foreground of my consciousness. Chopping onions, stir-frying greens, washing sweet potatoes—like breathing in and out, they allow my mind to settle into this moment.

It's the same practice when we are eating. We don't need to be in a particular mood or frame of mind to practice mindfulness while we eat. When we sit down with a plate of food, just like when we come into the kitchen or into meditation, we bring whatever is happening in our mind and heart with us. We hold it all with compassion, and we take our first bite in mindfulness. We savor the food and the givers—the earth, the sky, the chefs, and whomever else brought us this plate of nourishment. Then we take our next bite in mindfulness. And we continue to eat, bite by bite.

Whatever you are thinking or feeling is just one part of you, so don't leave any part of yourself behind when you come into the kitchen. Make room for surprises. If you bring your presence to the process of washing the rice, you might notice that a glimmer of joy is there along with your sadness or fear. As Zen Master Suzuki Roshi once said, "When you are in the dark, you don't know where you are going, but when you carefully feel your way along, where you find yourself will be okay."

Pancakes with Maple Syrup and/or Nut Butter
(vegan option)

I have probably cooked more pancakes than any other food in my life. To this day, certain young adults raised on my pancakes expect them to be served whenever they are staying at the house. Though I haven't always made the vegan version, it's very difficult to tell the difference between the vegan and non-vegan versions, especially when they are filled with blueberries or chocolate and drenched in delicious maple syrup.

INGREDIENTS:

1 tablespoon ground flax seed mixed into 3 tablespoons water;
   or 1 egg if not vegan

1 cup flour (unbleached white is nice, or ½ cup white and ½ cup wheat)

½ teaspoon baking soda

1 teaspoon baking powder

1 teaspoon turbinado sugar

1 cup almond milk (homemade recipe on **page 66**)

1 tablespoon apple cider vinegar

2 to 3 tablespoons grapeseed, coconut, walnut, or canola oil

vegan butter or almond butter

maple syrup

OPTIONAL:

blueberries, frozen or fresh

chocolate chips or cut up dark chocolate

METHOD:

Mix the flax seeds and water and let sit; or beat the egg.

Heat the oil on a griddle or large frying pan until water dropped onto the pan sizzles.

Sift together the dry ingredients.

Mix the vinegar into the almond milk.

Add the almond milk mixture into the dry ingredients and stir very gently, mixing only until all the flour has been absorbed. Some lumps are okay.

Scoop about ⅓ cup of batter and pour it gently onto the hot griddle or pan.

If adding blueberries or chocolate bits, sprinkle them into batter while on the griddle, amount to your liking.

Let cook until bottom is browned and batter starts to bubble. Flip and cook other side for several minutes until brown.

Spread finished pancakes with vegan butter or almond butter (adds protein), drizzle with maple syrup, and enjoy!

Makes approximately 10 smallish pancakes.

Stir-Fried Kale *(vegan)*

I tend to eat stir-fried greens nearly once every day. Sometimes I have them for breakfast, but most often at lunch or dinner. They are delicious, warming, and very healthy. Choose whichever greens are in season in your area. Some of my favorites are mustard greens (spicy), spinach (sweet), kale, chard, and collard greens (earthy). I usually only add salt because I find that additional seasoning tends to detract from the natural flavors. Make sure you use them before their impermanence starts to show and they turn yellow or brown!

INGREDIENTS:

　　1 bunch kale or other greens

　　2 to 3 tablespoons olive or other oil that can handle high heat

　　1 clove garlic, chopped (optional)

　　salt to taste, approximately ½ teaspoon

　　pepper to taste (optional)

METHOD:

Prepare the greens: wash and dry them. Take out the hard stalks that you
find at the end of mustard greens, chard, kale and collards. The roots
of spinach can be cut off, but the stems of spinach can be left on. Once
the fibrous stems are off, cut the greens cross-wise in slightly larger
than bite size pieces; they will shrink in the cooking.

Heat a large skilled over medium to high heat.

Add the oil to the skillet, and let it warm up until it just begins to smoke.

Add the garlic and stir for 30 seconds.

Add the greens, and immediately begin to stir with a wooden spoon.

Keep the greens moving as they begin to wilt. Spinach takes only 1 minute
to cook; some of the heartier greens may take several minutes. Don't
stop stirring until they are cooked.

Remove the skillet from the heat and add salt.

Serve immediately.

Serves approximately 4 to 5.

Microgreen Salad with Peanuts (vegan)

If you want to try enjoying vegetable chopping, make yourself this very simple yet delicious salad. You can throw pretty much anything in it, and the raisins, peanuts, and dressing give it a sweet, salty, and sour taste, which I find very satisfying.

INGREDIENTS:

> 8 to 10 large leaves of romaine lettuce
>
> 2 handfuls microgreens, if available
>
> ¼ cup sliced or chopped red onions
>
> Any other chopped vegetables that you like to eat raw such as carrots, cauliflower, radishes, or broccoli
>
> ¼ cup raisins (black or golden)
>
> ¼ cup salted peanuts, locally grown (if you happen to live near or in the South as I do)

METHOD:

Wash and rinse romaine and microgreens.

Chop or rip romaine leaves into bite-sized pieces. Add with microgreens to a large bowl.

Top with red onions, raisins, and peanuts.

Dress with Easy Oil and Vinegar dressing (see recipe on next page).

Serves 2 people as an appetizer or one hungry person.

Easy Oil and Vinegar Dressing *(vegan)*

INGREDIENTS:

- 3 tablespoons olive or other oil
- 1 tablespoon balsamic, fig, or other vinegar
- 2 tablespoons red onion minced into tiny pieces
- 1 clove garlic, minced
- 1 tablespoons agave syrup
- salt and pepper to taste

METHOD:

Mix all the dressing ingredients in an empty glass jar (or whisk with a fork in a bowl).

Cover the jar and shake gently until all ingredients are mixed, or about 5 times.

Let sit at room temperature for 30 minutes if possible, or you can use it immediately if need be. The longer the ingredients are together, the more flavorful the dressing will become.

Use on salad. Then cover and store the remainder in the refrigerator.

Serves 4 to 6.

Basic Sitting Meditation Practice

Sitting meditation is the foundation for learning mindfulness—the formal way we practice. It's like going to the gym to lift weights so you can be stronger in your daily life outside the gym. If you want to establish a strong mindfulness practice, I suggest that you practice a little bit each day, like five minutes, rather than trying to do longer meditations less often.

It's much easier to practice mindfulness alone on your cushion in a quiet spot. When we are around other people and in situations that are likely to upset us, it's harder to stay present. But the more we practice staying with our breathing in the moments on the cushion, the easier it will get for us to do it anywhere.

I think of mindfulness like I think of my yoga practice—I had to practice a long time before I could do a headstand. It's the same with mindfulness. Reading this book is a start, but in order to enjoy the benefits of meditation, you need to practice in real life.

A last note: On some days meditation will be smooth and easy and you will feel like you are really there with your breath. The next day your mind might be jumping all over the place. I've learned not to attach any importance to this, except to wonder, on days when my mind is really busy, if I am over-scheduled or anxious, and then I try to provide myself with some extra self-care that day. Our minds are a bit of a mystery, kind of like the weather. So try not to have too many expectations for how your meditation will be. Even after practicing for years, I'm still surprised each morning by the state of my mind.

1. Find a comfortable spot. If you have a timer (your smartphone will do) bring it with you.

2. Sit in an upright way (mostly so you won't fall asleep). If you're in a chair, let your feet be on the floor; if you're sitting cross-legged on a meditation cushion, be sure your legs are equally balanced (use a blanket or block to prop up one side if needed). I like to do sitting meditation in the kneeling position, straddling a meditation cushion; some people kneel using a Japanese meditation bench.

3. Set the timer for five minutes. You can close your eyes or let them gaze softly toward the floor. Your hands can rest on your knees or one on top of the other on your lap—whatever is comfortable for you.

4. Bring your attention to your breathing. Feel the movement of your body as your breath comes into your nose and out of your nose. You may notice that your belly and chest rise as you breathe in and fall as you breathe out. Just watch all of that without analyzing anything.

5. As soon as you notice that your mind has wandered and that you are no longer focused on the feeling of the breath, bring your mind back to your breath. Don't add any judgment, but if you do, notice that you judged—only notice, and don't add any new judgment (ad infinitum). Nothing is wrong or bad about your mind drifting; you're not trying to clear your mind of all thoughts—that would be impossible. You're just trying to develop the ability to bring your mind back to the present moment when it wanders away, like putting the frog back on the plate.

6. When the bell rings at the end of the meditation period, you can bow to yourself for taking the time to pause for a moment during the middle of your day for your own benefit. But don't forget that every moment on the cushion also benefits everyone you will come in contact with that day. Sitting like that will profit all beings everywhere.

7. Get up and go about your day. When you are standing in line somewhere, waiting for the bus, or walking the dogs, consider bringing your attention back to your breath or to your footsteps.

8. Repeat for the rest of your life.

Mindful Chocolate Ceremony

My co-teacher Linda and I created this ceremony to give the children who come to our Budding Yogis camp a taste of mindful eating. It is based on the tea ceremonies that take place at Plum Village, which are based on the classical tea ceremonies of Japan. Adults and children who practice this often say that it changes the way they eat and the way they think about food. Usually at least one person asks themselves the question, "What if I ate this way every day?"

1. Purchase chocolate that can be cut or broken into 1-inch pieces (or optionally, fruit, such as strawberries or oranges that can be served in bite-sized pieces).

2. Arrange enough chocolate (or fruit) and napkins for each person (including yourself) on a single tray. Add a few extra pieces of each item just in case. The tray should look very appealing, so consider adding a small fresh flower or other decoration.

3. Invite your group to sit in a circle. The circle should be close enough to pass the tray between individuals.

4. Explain to the group what you are about to do. Include the logistics (explained in numbers 4 to 6 below) as well as the intent, which is to be truly present for the food and the community.

At this point you can talk about mindfulness in general, mindful eating, what it means to you, and why you are practicing the chocolate ceremony. Let the participants know that they won't begin eating until everyone is served. When they do begin to eat, they can take their time and use all their senses to enjoy the chocolate—smell it, touch it, and finally, taste it. Once it is in their mouths, they can feel the texture and pay attention to how it melts, or chew it and notice how that feels. There is no right way to eat mindfully.

If you like, you can also invite people to consider where the food has come from: cacao trees, the people who farm it, the chocolatiers, the sunshine, rain, the people who packaged the chocolate, and even the one who stocked it at the grocery store. Be careful here not to encourage people to spend too much time thinking about the chocolate and forgetting to enjoy it!

5. Ask if anyone has any questions before you begin.

6. Ring the bell to indicate the formal beginning of the ceremony. From this point on, everything will happen in silence.

7. Pick up the tray and turn toward the person to your left. Smile and look into their eyes. That person bows to acknowledge your offering, and then takes a napkin and places it on their lap or on the ground in front of them. Then they choose a piece of chocolate (or a piece of fruit if there is one) and they place the food on the napkin. As you look at each other again, that person bows to you, you hand them the tray, and then bow to them. This completes the connection.

8. The person who received the tray, then turns to the person on their left and continues this process. The sharing continues this way in silence until the tray has come back to you. After you've all received your food, bowed, and taken the tray, you set the tray down in front of you or out of the way.

9. You then invite the bell to indicate that it is time to eat.

10. Everyone begins to sense the chocolate—looking at it, smelling it, and touching it before tasting it. Enjoy the chocolate and fruit slowly and thoroughly. When you see that at least half of the people have finished, invite the bell again to end the ceremony.

11. After the official ceremony is over, you can ask if there are any comments. At this point, the ceremony is over, and the tray can be passed again in an informal way, or placed in the center for people to pick up another piece when they would like.

12. Ask the participants to share with the group what it was like for them to eat like this. How did the chocolate taste differently than it might usually taste? What else did they notice about the food? What was it like to stay so focused and silent while passing and sharing the food?

13. When the time is up, you can invite the bell one last time, allowing everyone to bow to each other, stand up, and put away the leftovers.

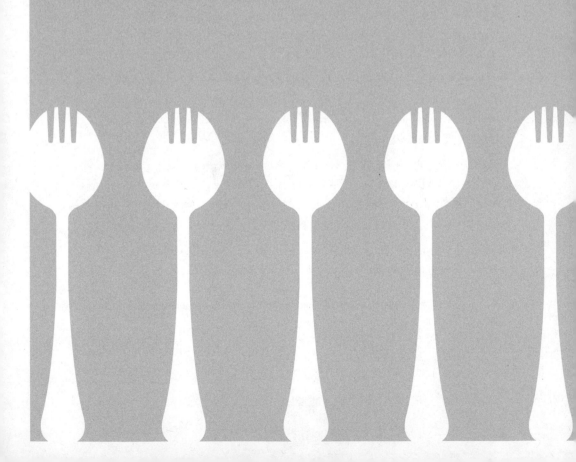

5.

PRESSURE COOKER

The monkey is reaching

For the moon in the water.

Until death overtakes him

He'll never give up.

If he'd let go the branch and

Disappear in the deep pool,

The whole world would shine

With dazzling pureness.

—HAKUIN EKAKU

It's late one Saturday afternoon and I am on my way home from dropping Jamie off at a play date on the other side of DC. I am alone for a few sweet moments, so naturally I make a mental tally of the kids. Where are they? Are they safe? Am I forgetting something I am supposed to be doing? What terrible parenting am I guilty of today?

I mumble to myself, like counting on my fingers, "Lucile is at home. I just dropped Jamie off at a play date, and Veronica went with a friend after soccer this morning… Let's see… What about Louie?" I pause, unable to remember where Louie is. Then it hits me. Oh shit. I left Louie at a birthday party four hours earlier. The party was over two hours ago. I turn the car around and head over to the birthday girl's house. I shamefully knock on the door, which opens to seven-year-old Louie playing happily with his friend in the living room. I am relieved to see him but incredulous. "Why didn't you call me?!" I inquire of the parents. "Oh, we figured you'd be here any minute." Louie and I leave. I have hit another parenting low.

LIKE A LOT OF FAMILIES, the schedule that we kept when our kids were school-age was completely ridiculous. Weekday afternoons were spent running between flute, soccer, baseball, piano lessons, Girl Scouts, and much more. Each weekend I sat at the computer and created two spreadsheets— one for Paul and one for me—of the kids' activities for which each of us was responsible. We both spent weekend days driving kids in different directions.

Being one of four had its risks. In addition to forgetting to pick up Louie from the birthday party, when he was an infant I left him in the car at a restaurant. Luckily, the friend I was meeting immediately asked me a question about some crayons that I had left in the car, and I remembered that the baby was there too. I ran the two blocks, opened the car, and pulled Louie out. I went back into the restaurant trying to act natural amidst the strange looks from my friends and the waiter.

I often fretted about the craziness of our lives, and I spent a lot of time ruminating about the ways in which I could or should be doing it better. I began doing ten to twenty minutes of sitting meditation each morning, but I had to get up at 5:30 a.m. to find a moment of peace and quiet before the bedlam of the family day began. Even still, my mind was filled with so many "if onlys." If only my husband would cook or clean. If only Jamie, Veronica, and Lucile would have been on the same travel soccer teams, rather than three different ones. If only Louie wanted to play soccer instead of the guitar. If only my parents lived closer to us. Like The Three Bears, it always seemed that there was a family state that would be "just right" if only we could find it. My to-do lists spanned multiple pages in my journal and included items like "TANGO!" alongside "Pick up new strings for Veronica's violin."

I Ate the Whole Mango

One day I was eating a mango at my kitchen table. It was delicious. My daughter Jamie, who especially loves mangoes, was sitting in the other room studying for her high school exams. As I savored the first half of my mango, I thought about her sitting in the living room and how she would really enjoy having some of it. I considered taking the second half to her. I thought about how happy she would be to have it, and that made me smile.

Then I ate the rest of the mango. I ate the rest of the mango because as a working mother of four young kids, I needed some nurturing myself. I wasn't ready to be generous in that moment because I wasn't taking care of my own needs—and taking care of ourselves also benefits those around us. This truth was clearly articulated on a sweatshirt that Veronica gave me many years ago. It said, "If mama ain't happy, ain't nobody happy."

Hungry Ducks

I wish I had been able to share the mango with Jamie. And I wish that I had been able to carve out more time, or at least mental space, to take care of my own needs. In a training I took with nonviolent communication teacher

Marshall Rosenberg, he told a story about a woman, like me, who was tired of making dinner for her family every night. Like me, she was overwhelmed with all the things she was doing and was becoming resentful because cooking was one of the things she didn't want to do.

I thought I was obligated to do certain things—that some things were not a choice. Rosenberg believes differently. He says that everyone benefits when we make decisions from a place of choice, like when a small child chooses to feed some hungry ducks. He says that we should never do anything that we can't do with that kind of joy, because if we do things out of guilt, obligation, or fear, then someone—maybe us, maybe the person we are doing it for, or maybe a complete stranger—will be punished by the fallout later. I have heard him say, "Whenever you make a request of someone, hand them a little card that says this on it: 'Please do as I requested only if you can do so with the joy of a little child feeding a hungry duck.'"

This woman, resentful about making dinner every night for her family, told her story at Rosenberg's workshop. Rosenberg advised her to stop making dinner. So she did. A few weeks later, her son and her husband showed up at one of his workshops. Rosenberg was worried that they were going to be furious and tell him off. But instead they came to thank him. They explained that the woman was much easier to live with and much happier, which made them all much happier too.

I loved that story! It brought tears to my eyes to imagine how much relief she must have felt giving up her burden. But I also thought, "What a crock of shit." My family would not be celebrating if I stopped making dinner or cleaning up after them. And then who would cook? Certainly not my husband—unless we wanted to eat cheesy eggs or fondue every night—and not my kids. They were too busy running around between activities and doing mounds of homework to have learned anything about cooking from me.

Even though I wasn't sure how it would work, I wove Rosenberg's teaching into my mindfulness practice and began to examine how I was really feeling about each of the activities in my life, rather than continuing to do them out of habit or obligation. When I did that, I discovered that I no longer felt good about cooking meat for my family. I actually loved cooking, but I wanted to cook only a single dinner each night—a vegetarian one. One night, as I was cleaning chicken breasts and pulling off the slimy fascia, I suddenly knew that was it. I couldn't do it anymore. Once I made that change, I felt tremendously relieved. Cooking vegetarian food was more compatible with my intentions. Paul and the kids weren't thrilled about the change, but the kids were old enough to buy their own food or snacks outside the house, and no one was surprised about my declaration. From then on we ate only vegetarian food when I cooked.

Like Mother, Like Daughter

Lucile was aware of her appearance from a young age. She was tiny, with long wavy brown hair and large, almond-shaped brown eyes. She carried the Armenian genes and was the shortest in most of her classes. All through elementary school she took ballet, which unfortunately taught her that a tall, thin body was the most desirable shape.

She was also a pleaser and took other people's comments to heart, though she rarely showed it. On the night before her first day of kindergarten, I came upstairs and found her on a stepladder in front of the linen closet. She had her two "blankies," which she adored and took everywhere she went, in her hands. I asked her what she was doing, and she said that she didn't need her blankies anymore since she was big enough to go to school. She shoved them onto the highest shelf she could reach and climbed down, acting as if it were no big deal. (We retrieved them a few days later.) I worried that if Lucile focused on how she "should" act or look, she would lose the ability to tap into her own inner sense of rightness.

In the same way that an alcoholic is almost always the first to finish her glass of wine, food addicts are often the first to clean our plates or go for seconds because we are the least attentive to what we are eating. My dad had been that way, I had been that way, and now Lucile was finding herself experiencing the same thing. When she visited friends' houses (where they allowed more junk food) she would often eat way too many cupcakes or pretzels.

Lucile also had the habit of isolating herself when she was feeling down. Many mornings she was too "tired" to go to school, and many more days I went to school to pick her up because she had a headache or was simply unwell. We now know that some part of this was due to her then-undiagnosed food allergies, but it made me sad to see how powerless I was to prevent my pattern of avoiding feelings from being passed down to her. Paul and I encouraged her to see a therapist who suggested that Lucile's unhappiness was likely stemming from the family system, so my husband and I also began couples therapy.

Veronica was actually the tallest girl in many of her classes. She was the opposite of Lucile, blonde with a strong athletic build. Her twin, Jamie, was a few inches shorter and had a smaller bone structure. The biggest of the three girls (she was taller than Lucile by the age of six) Veronica was always embarrassed about her size. When she was ten and at a normal weight, her soccer coach (a young man) told her that she needed to lose weight in order to run faster. It confirmed her worst fears and she was devastated. She quit the team and began the familiar pattern of shame and overeating.

Veronica left notes on my computer some mornings that I would find when I returned home from walking the kids to their neighborhood elementary school. They said things like, "Dear Mom, I am so unhappy. I have no friends and I am fat. Please help me." Reading these notes made my heart break. I could see that she had so much suffering inside. Paul and I helped Veronica change schools, get educational and psychological testing, and therapy, and even sent her to a weight loss camp, along with her brother (who asked to go there because of his own awareness of his eating addictions), but nothing mitigated her underlying pain. Going on a mindfulness retreat, which we did every year, was a respite for her because it was a chance to be with whatever was arising, in a container of friendship and support, but it didn't change her day-to-day suffering.

When Lucile accepted our suggestion that she go into treatment for her eating disorder, I had to accept that my dysfunctional eating habits and history had an effect on our family. I was in therapy at the time, and I said to my therapist, "I don't want my kids to suffer, and I don't want to pass any of my messed-up eating habits on to them." "Well," she said, "you already have." I could barely breathe.

When I visited Lucile at her treatment center, she took me to her Anorexics and Bulimics Anonymous (ABA) Twelve-Step program. It was similar to other twelve-step meetings I had attended. The ten or so of us (all women) sat in a circle reading from the ABA blue book and sharing our experiences. Being an outsider to this particular program of recovery, I felt slightly superior.

Near the end of the meeting, the leader asked if anyone had an anniversary. Had anyone been free from bingeing and purging for one day? Someone raised her hand, and she was given a little blue chip. The leader asked about two-day anniversaries, then three-day anniversaries, and so on. When she asked about one-week anniversaries, Lucile stood up to get her chip. I was so proud of her. The leader moved from weeks to months and then to year anniversaries, delivering them more rapidly as the lengths of time increased.

When she asked if anyone had been binge- and purge-free for twenty years, my stomach completely turned over. It suddenly hit me that I was absolutely a member of this community of recovery—I just hadn't acknowledged it to Lucile or myself until then. It had always been her problem or Veronica's problem. Even though I had been meditating for nine years at this point, I still hadn't fully owned my past eating disorder.

I was almost too ashamed to raise my hand and to let Lucile see that I was as wounded as she was. But in that split second, I decided to be as vulnerable as she had, and I reached out to receive my little red chip. It was a humbling remembrance of the suffering I shared with my daughter, and I keep my red chip on my altar as a reminder.

All those years, I had tried to make healthy choices and hide my own preoccupations with food and weight, and yet here we were with one bulimic daughter and another daughter coming into a destructive binge-eating habit. Veronica's food issues had been growing as a result of her anxiety and depression, and she was rarely happy. By the time she reached high school she was secretly binge eating at night. Rather than feel my sadness and accept that I had almost no control over their suffering, I shot myself with the second arrow of self-blame. I convinced myself that their difficulties were all my fault. This thinking kept me preoccupied with myself and my mistakes, which not only caused me terrible guilt, but also distanced me from my girls and their actual experiences and seeing how I might help.

One night, I was sobbing in bed, my head against Paul's chest, feeling like everything I had done was wrong. I was thinking about their pain and how it was all a result of my bad parenting. Paul pulled his head back, tipped it slightly, and stared at me with a look of disbelief. "Do you really think that Lucile's eating disorder is all your fault?" I nodded. Then he asked, "Do you think all of our family's issues are your fault too?" I answered, "Yes!" The look of disbelief in Paul's eyes was like a crack in the armor of my self-blame. Maybe it wasn't all my fault after all.

Although blaming my children's problems on myself seemed altruistic, it wasn't selfless or helpful at all. It suggested that they had no agency in their own lives—that I was the puppet master pulling all the strings. It also denied the truth of interdependence. Our kids had many other important influences in their lives, including their dad, their aunts and uncles, their siblings, their peers, and society. Blaming myself for all of my children's difficulties was just another second arrow. But ignoring or disowning their suffering was not going to be helpful either. I had to find a middle way.

Thinking about who is to blame, what we should have done (cognitive behavioral therapy calls this "shoulding" on ourselves and others), and what would have happened "if only" we had done something different isn't just about being more mindful. Mindfulness can even become another "should" or "if only" ("if only I were more mindful, I'd be happy"). True mindfulness goes beyond all these concepts and sees into the reality of just what is.

Spending our time ruminating over who did what when, who should have done what when, and if only things were different causes at least three big problems in our lives: 1. We miss what's really happening in our lives. While we are inside our heads figuring out who was right or wrong, or who won, we miss the beauty of the tulip garden next door, the feeling of our daughter's hand inside of ours, and the sound of the snow melting off our roof, not to mention the taste of our food. 2. We aren't happy. Think about a moment when you have been the happiest. I guarantee it wasn't during a session of mental gymnastics. Our happiest moments are when we give and receive love or experience the fleeting pleasures of a hot bath, a heartfelt interaction, a star-filled sky, or good sex. 3. We are alone. No one else inhabits our mind except us. The more time we spend alone up there, the less time we spend with other people. When we are blaming and ruminating, we can't reach out to support anyone else, and we can't feel it when someone tries to reach us. Being cut off from our senses is the loneliest place on earth.

Talking Tofurky

Every year since my grandmother died, my favorite cousin, Mark, has invited us over for Thanksgiving at his house. I love going to his house, reconnecting with the extended family, and enjoying a festive meal—everything but the turkey. When I first stopped eating meat, I ate the potatoes, dressing, cheesy cabbage, salad, and pie, and just skipped the turkey. I got some rolled eyes, but no one seemed to care. But when I started bringing the Tofurky and asking for space in the oven to cook it, tensions rose.

I'll admit it, I was annoying. I made the full Tofurky meal with the included "dressing" and "gravy," and I made sure the Tofurky got passed around, telling people how delicious it was. I was oblivious to the dirty looks and smirks passed between cousins when I wasn't looking. I didn't find out that the family was irritated with me until I read something my cousin wrote online. In it, he suggested that the vegetarians and vegans he knew were pushy and selfish (I might have been the only one he knew!) and that he thought we should stop asking for special consideration and instead be grateful for what we were offered. I was shocked and hurt.

On my next retreat, I complained to my friend, a longtime mindfulness student and twenty-five-year vegetarian. She asked me matter-of-factly, "Why don't you just eat the turkey?" But I didn't want to eat it, and I didn't think, as a good mindfulness practitioner, I was "supposed" to eat meat. My intention, based on The Five Mindfulness Trainings, was not to destroy life. But I also had the intention to speak mindfully and not in ways that would case relationships to break. How could I manage both of these intentions?

Sister Chan Khong, a close student of Thich Nhat Hanh for the last fifty years, says, "I have met people who cannot be vegetarian because of medical reasons, but who respect life more than many vegetarians. Some vegetarians are too extreme and are unkind to those who cannot give up meat-eating. I am more comfortable with a meat-eater than with an extreme vegetarian who is filled with self-righteousness."

A friend of mine summed it up when she said, "Pass the turkey, not the judgment." The next time I went to Thanksgiving at Mark's house, I decided not to bring a Tofurky and to eat in a way that didn't create any discord. I don't particularly like the taste of turkey, so I didn't eat it. But I didn't make a big deal out of it, and I did my best to eat everything else with gratitude.

I have found that mindfulness isn't a solo self-improvement project, but rather a way to stay more engaged in the world in which we find ourselves. Being mindful of one thing, like what or how we eat, can easily create another bad habit as a consequence if we aren't careful. Mindfulness means we practice bringing awareness and compassion to whatever or whoever is in front of us in any particular moment, whether it's the turkey, the Tofurky, or your favorite cousin.

Coming of Age

When Lucile moved on to junior high school, I decided that our kids needed to have a coming-of-age ritual. Rather than have a ceremony, we decided that each child would go on an overseas trip with only the same-gendered parent to a less commercially developed country. The trip was created to challenge each child's comfort zone in specific ways: They were exposed to completely different foods, languages they didn't know, and people lacking the many privileges that they enjoyed. They still had a parent with them, but they were taken out of their comfort zone for a while.

I loved the simplicity of life and food on these trips, and each time I returned home, I vowed to modify our typical American diet to include more fresh food and less junk. I wanted to solve our family's growing problems with eating. Every time I tried this, I got laughed at and ignored. No desserts? Okay, we'll buy candy. Fresh vegetables? Not gonna eat them. Eventually, I gave up and we all went back to our old eating habits.

Each time I returned from a trip I thought I had the secret to solving my (and our) dysfunctional eating habits, with more "if onlys." If only we didn't eat dessert, none of us would have problems with eating. If only I don't eat meat, I won't be harming anyone.

There's nothing wrong with practicing intentions. But what I had to learn was that there is no way to get it right. I'm ashamed to admit that I wanted to feel smug. I wanted to get mindfulness right. What I really wanted was to get life right.

Knowing the truth that the world is impermanent and that we are all interconnected, means that if we lean on any concept too heavily, we will fall. Norman Fishcher tells the story of a time when Zen Master Suzuki Roshi was traveling with one of his more accomplished students, who was a strict vegetarian. They stopped at a restaurant to have a meal, and when the waiter came, the student ordered a salad. To the student's shock, Suzuki Roshi ordered a hamburger. The student revered the Roshi, so he didn't say anything about the hamburger. When the food arrived, Suzuki Roshi took a bite of the hamburger, pushed it in front of his student, and took the student's salad.[5] I don't think Suzuki Roshi was implying that everyone should eat meat. I think he wanted to remind his student not to cling too tightly to any one concept—like vegetarianism—because nothing we do or don't do will make us immune to difficulties. Even if we had the perfect diet, were friendly and compassionate to everyone, gave away all our belongings, and lived like a monk, we wouldn't get to skip the suffering.

To grasp onto concepts of right and wrong is just another way to stay caught in our minds. When we loosen our grip on what we think we know, we fall headlong into real life—full of paradox and imperfection. It's within this very life of paradox and imperfection, cooked and eaten with a generous dash of gentle mindfulness, that we will find our bliss.

As the Sufi poet Rumi said, "Out beyond ideas of wrongdoing and right-doing, there is a field. I'll meet you there."

Washing Dishes

Like trying to eat the right foods or keep my email inbox empty, maintaining a perfect kitchen is impossible too. Just as you start the dishwasher, someone brings a pile of dirty dishes. Just when you turn off the kitchen light at night, someone flicks it back on and starts preparing a snack. The dog food gets spilled, a glass is broken. It's useless to try to control it too tightly. The kitchen is the heart of our home and so it's always been well lived-in. I liked to start cooking a meal with a clean kitchen, though, so sometimes I spent half an hour cleaning up before starting to cook.

As humor writer Erma Bombeck once said, "Housework, if you do it right, will kill you." I wanted to find a way to apply my new mindfulness practice to the household situation. Between the growing business of the yoga studio and my family, I never had time to pause except during my morning meditation. Then I discovered that I didn't have to wait to sit on my cushion; I could practice mindfulness *while* I was cooking and cleaning.

When I washed the dishes, I tried to remember that the water was warm and that, if I slowed down, it was kind of like giving a baby a bath. Thich Nhat Hanh says, "There are two ways to wash the dishes. The first is to wash the dishes in order to have clean dishes, and the second is to wash the dishes in order to wash the dishes." Even if we are in a hurry, we can bring some mindfulness to our dishwashing. When we do that, we can have a moment of ease right in the middle of our hectic life.

The same is true with every task that we do. We can be mindful of driving, typing, speaking, vacuuming, or cooking, just by bringing our awareness to the sensations we are feeling in the moment. It's not about making our work more perfect (though being mindful may indeed improve the quality of our work), but about really living our lives.

I copied a mindfulness poem on my bathroom mirror in dry-erase marker so I would see it as soon as I got to the bathroom each morning. It said, "Waking up this morning I smile. Twenty-four brand-new hours are before me. I vow to live fully in each moment, and to look at all beings with the eyes of compassion." Some mornings, I didn't even make it to the mirror before I was lost in my mind worrying about the events of the day.

Many mornings, I opened my eyes and my first awareness was the stench of dog poop floating up from the family room below. Our aging poodle had the misfortune of getting diarrhea whenever he was fed from the table, and instead of making a pile near the door, he walked while he pooped on every square foot of rug in the house. On other mornings, I might be awakened by a feverish child or by the sound of someone throwing up in another room. It wasn't always easy to look at certain beings with the eyes of compassion, but I was trying.

Le Food

One summer, after our now-annual retreat to Plum Village, in France, my son Louie and I made a stop in Paris for a few days. He was fourteen at the time, and was immersed in skateboard culture—he had even brought his board from Washington, DC, to France. We did some sightseeing and had lunch, and then he asked me whether he could visit some local skate shops on his own. I was so relaxed and happy after the retreat that I said, "Yeah, sure. Let's meet back here at this park at 4:00 p.m."

At 2:00 p.m., I started to think about what he was doing. By 3:00, I was panicking. What was I thinking? I could barely find this park again myself, so how would a fourteen-year-old boy find it? And why would I let him ride his longboard around the busy Paris streets? Most important, what would I do if he didn't show up at 4:00? Neither of us spoke French, and neither of us had cell phones. Luckily, he appeared right at 4:00, and I breathed a huge sigh of relief.

While he survived those few hours in Paris alone, they changed our lives. On our last morning in Paris, Louie looked at me and said sincerely, "Mom, will you leave me here?" He was smitten. Almost as soon as we landed in DC, he began applying for student exchange programs in France, and just after Christmas that year, he flew to Rennes in Brittany, in northwest France.

Louie was placed with a wonderful family that we have gotten to know well over the years since he came home. His host father was Jean-Luc, a tall, athletic businessman who had once lived in Indiana for two years for his work. Jean-Luc would say to Louie, "Okay, we spoke English in the morning, this afternoon we only speak French." His host mother, Nelly, was a calm, easy-going woman with short red hair and a constant smile who worked full-time as a hairdresser.

Louie, who had only studied French for a few months, finished tenth-grade year in a huge French public high school where he made lots of friends. His French family, especially Nelly, had a very different approach to preparing and eating meals than I did, which he told me about when he came home and which I experienced firsthand when our family visited Rennes the following year.

On a typical day, Nelly made dinner for the family: Jean-Luc and her two children (plus Louie when he lived with them). Nelly looked forward to the process of preparing a meal, even after she'd been on her feet as a hairdresser all day. The evening meal was the highlight of their day, and both Nelly and Jean-Luc considered what they would prepare. For Nelly, cooking was a chance to shift gears, express her creativity, and focus on the sensual pleasures of the food.

When we were in Rennes, Nelly cooked as she normally would. She made a simple meal that included sliced cantaloupe, crepes filled with ham and cheese, steamed carrots and potatoes, sliced baguette, and a store-bought cake for dessert. It wasn't what she cooked, but her energy around food that struck me as so unusual. When she maneuvered around the kitchen, she seemed both relaxed and focused. She seemed to be, as a popular song says, dancing like nobody was watching. She invited me to step out back with her to have a cigarette between putting veggies in the steamer and cutting a melon. Jean-Luc poured wine, and the three children spent time catching up with each other and texting their friends. I'd guess that Nelly didn't find every meal this relaxing, but she didn't give nasty looks or emit resentment in the kitchen the way I often did.

What was Nelly's secret? She didn't have more time or energy than I did. Her kitchen was smaller than ours and had fewer cooking gadgets, and she had about the same access to fresh food. But Nelly had much less internal chatter about cooking. When she was cooking, she cooked. She wasn't preoccupied with other things. And although her simple cheese plate looked lovely, she wasn't preoccupied with our judgment of her finished product while she was cooking.

Food was a stress-free pleasure in this French family. Making dinner wasn't a last-minute rush job done grudgingly for others, it was a family activity integrated into each day. Nelly cooked at her own pace, never rushing. There was no firm time for the beginning or end of the meal the way there was in our home. As long as dinner was done before bedtime, it was okay. Cooking and eating were the only events of the evening—an enjoyable way to unwind from their busy days and reconnect with family, not simply a chore to get done.

In contrast, I was always trying to squeeze dinner into our schedule. At our house, it was as if dinner was a last-minute surprise each day ("Oh shit! It's dinnertime!"), even though this event happened 365 days a year without fail. I worried that we were eating too late or too early, the kids wouldn't have time to do their homework, my husband would be late for dinner, the food wouldn't be healthy/vegetarian/local/special enough, and there wouldn't be enough or there would be too much waste. Watching

Nelly prepare a meal, I saw that because of my food issues, I had never really been calm and comfortable around food.

I saw a similar comfort around food during our trip to Vietnam. The laywomen associated with each temple whipped up vegetarian feasts for hundreds of temple guests. They needed little space and used the simplest equipment and implements. They wouldn't even have known what to do with all the gadgets and counter space in my kitchen back home. They cooked delicious feasts in huge pots on open fires or gas rings that were set on the earth outside the temple kitchen. They sat on tiny plastic chairs, squatted, or stood bending over the pots as they stirred, watched, and added ingredients, and once in a while exchanged a few words with one another. Clearly comfort with food is not dependent on such privileges as having food processors, pasta makers, and a six-burner stove.

During these and other travels, I saw over and over again how much more comfortable people in other cultures were with their food. I witnessed firsthand that it was possible to live without the angst I generally had around food. In Morocco, men cooked and ate recently slaughtered animals, while squatting and chatting at the side of the road. In the rainforest, whatever came out of the river that day was happily grilled, shared, and eaten.

I also noticed that these other cultures ate only at certain prescribed times of the day. There was no snacking in the car, on the camel, or while hiking. In each of these places, eating was a ritual act, with a clear beginning, middle, and end. It started with a toast or a prayer, and finished with a full belly. I thought to myself, if hundreds of millions of people can have a more straightforward and less-fraught relationship to food, I can too.

Just knowing this allowed me to begin to transform. Whenever I noticed that I was stressing myself out in the kitchen by ignoring the sensual pleasures of cooking and the privilege of having food to eat, drowning my feelings in eating, or thinking I wasn't doing it "right," I paused and said hello to these habits. I made space between my experiences and these habitual patterns of reacting and thinking.

No Emergencies

Even when we have a lot to do in our lives, we can still find ways to approach the kitchen with ease. When we practice simply cooking the food in front of us, rather than engaging in thoughts about the past and worries about the future, we bring more joy to those we cook for and to ourselves. My friend Eve says that mindful cooking offers her a "daily source of joy." This reminds me of the lyrics to the verse of a Plum Village song:

Happiness is here and now,
I have dropped my worries.
Somewhere to go, something to do,
but I don't need to hurry.

Yoga teacher Judith Lasater, perhaps best known for her promotion of restorative yoga for relaxation, once told a class, "The only emergency is when someone is almost dying. If they are dead already, it's not an emergency, and if they aren't almost dying, it's not an emergency." Luckily, most of us in the developed world aren't experiencing those kinds of emergencies, but we often act as though we are. When we take the time to pause, see things in perspective, and enjoy a moment, we allow our brains to absorb positive feelings, to remember what's right and not just what's wrong—and to lay the groundwork for even more positive moments. As I have heard several mindfulness teachers say, "Don't just do something—sit there."

Given the human negativity bias, we can achieve balance by becoming experts in generating joy. It takes somewhere between twelve and thirty seconds of experiencing a positive state of mind for it to sink in and change our brain chemistry. That's less time than you might spend sitting at a red light. As Glen Schneider describes in his little book *Ten Breaths to Happiness*, the time it takes to breathe in and out ten times is all you need to fully absorb a pleasant experience.

It takes only twelve seconds to let even the smallest pleasant situations— like the way the sun is coming in our kitchen window, or the smell of the apple we are slicing—truly sink in. Those extra seconds spent in awareness while cooking a dish will eventually sensitize your brain to notice more pleasant moments in the kitchen and elsewhere.

Moreover, even if it's not our natural state, we can learn to relax in the kitchen and at the table. When we are relaxed, our parasympathetic nervous system sends more blood to our digestive organs. Neurobiologist Hanson says that even simple things like relaxing our tongue while eating can help move us into the parasympathetic nervous system and allow us to digest our food more fully and feel better while we do it.

But when we are stressed or rushed, our sympathetic nervous system activates and draws energy away from those organs to prepare us for a fight, flight, or freeze response. I remember feeling this happen a few years ago at a noodle restaurant Paul and I frequent; we hadn't been there in a while, and Paul, who doesn't normally go out for lunch, felt rushed. I said something about his bad mood, which got us going, and by the time my dish arrived—my favorite Drunken Noodles with Spicy Basil Sauce and Tofu—I was annoyed and fighting back my tears. But rather than using my meal to numb my feelings, I stayed aware of my inner pain while I took my first bite. I noticed that my stomach was in knots and my noodles tasted like anger.

Thich Nhat Hanh has often said that if you are thinking about your problems when you eat, then you are eating your problems. When I wasn't mindful, I covered up my discomfort with food, but when I stayed present with my feelings, I couldn't finish my noodles. I took them home and ate them after I took care of my anger. Although I still felt upset and a bit nauseous when I left the restaurant, I was pleased to have paid close attention to what my body really wanted.

I left the restaurant that day reminded of how important it is to be mindful not just of what we eat, but of the conversations we have while we are eating. I think of it as mouth yoga—being mindful of everything that goes in and out of my mouth. Since dinner is often the only time of day when our family sits down together, I want to be mindful of what happens. If you habitually use the dinner hour as a time to bring up difficulties, worries, or have family quarrels, children may begin to avoid dinner or worse, develop digestive issues. It might be more productive to bring up concerns before or after dinner so that your shared meal can be a time of positive connection and pleasure—and a time to slow down and relax at the table and enjoy being together.

Over the years, inspired by the countries I've visited, our family has developed ways of making our meals more relaxed. With Nelly as a role model, I try to let meal preparation be the main event, not just a way to get food on the table. It doesn't always work, but as Mark Twain said, "Habit is habit, and not to be flung out of the window by any man, but coaxed downstairs one step at a time."

Ritual

Since our kids were small, we've begun our meal by holding hands and saying or singing grace, then taking a minute of silence. As they got older we came up with other fun rituals for dinnertime, like "singing our day" (see page 143). Sometimes we each took turns renaming the art on the walls surrounding our dining room table. These funny rituals helped a baseline-anxious family relax and laugh.

As years passed, the kids started to mock the moment of silence and the singing, so we just shared about our day. During their teenage years, when they were angry, one of them might refuse to hold hands, say grace, or even speak. Once in a great while, someone would miss family dinner, and instead eat something in his or her room. During those difficult years, I often got discouraged and wondered if all of our dinner rituals had been pointless after all.

But just like in meditation, in the best of times we sat together, and in the worst of times we sat together. When Jamie's kitten died suddenly, we sat down at the table. When Lucile and her boyfriend broke up, we sat down and ate together. When Veronica won the distinguished religion student award, we sat down as a family. Even on the days when none of us could stand being together, we sat down and ate dinner together. By the end of dinner, even if we were feuding, at least we felt somewhat reconnected.

On nights when I was impatient, or when we had only fifteen minutes to eat, I might try skipping grace, but one of us always reached out to take hands, and the singing would begin. We often had the kids' friends over to eat, and most hadn't experienced a big family dinner with so much interaction. They loved it.

An interesting study done at the University of Minnesota in 2013 showed that even the smallest rituals can make a difference in our eating experience.[6] In the study, each subject was given a candy bar to eat. Half the subjects were asked to simply eat it in a relaxed way; the others were asked to perform a small ritual before they ate it. Scientists discovered that subjects who did the ritual—breaking the candy in half, unwrapping one half and eating it, then unwrapping the second half and eating it—rated the chocolate as better-tasting and savored it more than the subjects who were instructed to simply relax before eating it.

Even today, when Paul and I eat together alone (which is most of the time now that the kids have moved out), we still hold hands and say or sing grace, or take some time to sit in silence. At the very minimum we say, "Bon appetit!" and clink glasses. Even when we have dinner guests, we observe some kind of small ritual. Holding hands and saying grace signals to us that its time to relax, taste our food, and enjoy everyone's company. It marks the beginning of a sacred time.

I have recently begun to practice a ritual when I am beginning to cook as well. When I come into the kitchen, I pause and breathe in and out slowly one time, before doing anything else. As I begin, either by washing my hands or taking things out of the cupboard or refrigerator, I think to myself, "May whatever I make benefit those who eat it." It's simple, but it changes my attitude from one of being hurried and goal-oriented to one of mindfulness and contributing.

Simple Chickpea Stew *(vegan)*

Although it's not as special as the delicious Vietnamese herbed soups and stews we had in Plum Village, this one is pretty good and very simple to make. You can whip this up for dinner in only a few minutes.

INGREDIENTS:

  2 tablespoons oil (I like to use olive oil.)

  ½ onion, peeled and diced

  ½ teaspoon of salt

  1 teaspoon garlic powder

  ½ teaspoon pepper

  1 teaspoon paprika

  ¼ teaspoon cayenne

  2 teaspoons cumin

  15 ounces fire-roasted tomatoes (1 can)

  1 cup spinach or kale (frozen or fresh)

  2 cups cooked chickpeas

METHOD:

In a medium-sized saucepan, heat the oil.

Once it's hot, add the onion and sauté until clear and beginning to brown.

Add tomatoes, including juice, and the spices.

Cook just until it boils, then reduce heat to simmer and add greens and chickpeas.

Cover and simmer for 10 to 15 minutes.

Serve over the grain of your choice.

Serves 4.

Beets on Hummus *(vegan)*

My friend Gisele Theriault introduced me to this delicious beet salad.

INGREDIENTS FOR HUMMUS:

   2 cups edamame (fresh or frozen), shelled

   juice of 2 lemons

   4 cloves of garlic, peeled and coarsely chopped

   2½ tablespoons tahini

   1 tablespoon olive, or similar, oil

   salt to taste

INGREDIENTS FOR BEETS:

   1 tablespoon olive, or similar, oil

   4 beets, peeled and cut into 1-inch squares

   ¼ cup roasted pine nuts (to roast, heat small pan on medium heat,
      add pine nuts, and stir or flip until lightly browned)

   1 cup arugula or arugula sprouts

   pumpkin seed oil (optional)

METHOD FOR HUMMUS:

Defrost edamame.

Combine the edamame, juice of 1 lemon, garlic, tahini, 1 tablespoon of
   oil, and salt in a blender or food processor, and blend until smooth and
   fully mixed.

Add water or extra olive oil as you blend to reach the desired consistency.

METHOD FOR BEETS:

Boil the beets for 20 minutes in water, then let cool to room temperature.

Squeeze the juice of 1 lemon onto the beets and toss.

Spread the hummus on the plate, about ½ inch thick.

Drizzle the pumpkin seed oil on the hummus if desired.

Put the beets on top of the hummus.

Circle the dish with arugula and sprinkle on the pine nuts over the top.

Serves 4.

St. Mary's Red Lentil Patties *(vegan)*

I learned to make this dish from the Armenian women at St. Mary Armenian Apostolic Church in Washington, DC. During Lent they have an annual bazaar and food festival at which they serve only vegetarian food, including rice pilaf, cheese boreg (triangles), lentil soup, hummus, and these amazing red lentil patties. One year I decided to see if my Armenian genes would help me learn to make some of the delicious dishes. I volunteered to come the morning before the bazaar to make hundreds of lentil patties. It was great fun, and now I make these patties for my family and myself whenever I like. There was no written recipe, so I scribbled notes when I wasn't forming patties, and adapted it for a few hundred fewer people, replacing the butter with Earth Balance.

INGREDIENTS:

    2 cups dry red lentils

    2 cups fine bulgur

    4 cups water

    ½ onion, finely chopped

    4 teaspoons cumin

    1 teaspoon garlic powder

    1 teaspoon cayenne

    2 teaspoons salt

    2 teaspoons pepper

    2 tablespoons olive oil, Earth Balance, or other vegan margarine

GARNISH:

    paprika

    parsley (about ½ cup)

    scallions (I use about 10.)

METHOD:

Place the lentils in a large pot with the 4 cups of water.

Bring to a boil, and then reduce heat to simmer.

Cover, and simmer until lentils are soft, around 15 to 20 minutes.

Heat 1 to 2 tablespoons olive oil or vegan margarine in a frying pan over medium heat.

Add onions and cook until onions are soft and translucent, stirring constantly.

Add bulgur and onions to the lentils.

Turn off heat, add spices, and stir.

When the mixture is cool enough to be handled, mold into patties about the size of a small burger, and place on serving plate.

Garnish with paprika, parsley, and scallions.

Serve at room temperature.

Makes about 16 to 20 patties.

Baked Pears (vegan)

This dessert, like those we had in Morocco, Ecuador, and Greece, isn't too sweet. You can add more maple syrup if you'd like, but if the pears are ripe, I find it sweet enough without any syrup at all.

INGREDIENTS:

    4 pears, peeled and cored

    1 tablespoon vegan margarine (I use Earth Balance) per pear

    1 tablespoon maple syrup per pear

    salt

    cinnamon

METHOD:

Preheat oven to 350 degrees.

Place pears on baking sheet with a few sprinkles of water.

Place 1 tablespoon of margarine on each pear.

Drizzle 1 tablespoon of maple syrup on each pear.

Add a dash of salt and a sprinkle of cinnamon on each pear.

Bake until pears are soft all the way through, about 10 minutes.

Serves 4.

Mindful Rituals for the Family Meal

Sitting down together for a family meal is a wonderful way to reconnect parents who have been working and kids who have been in school all day. Connecting can be supported in any number of ways. Here are a few of my favorite family-tested dinner activities:

1. Sing your day. Each person sings about their day in whatever form they like. Kids (or parents) can stand on their chair to sing for dramatic effect. Acting out important parts is also allowed. Singing lightens things up; teenagers are less likely to feel they're being forced to report on their day, and everyone has an opportunity to glimpse each others' worlds.

2. Create a gratitude grace. Before starting the meal, ask each person to say one thing that they have been grateful for that day.

3. Start the meal with one to two minutes of silent eating to allow everyone to really taste the food. Each evening a different family member can be the "bell master" who keeps time and rings the bell when silent time begins and ends.

4. A bell or talking stick can be used to pass around the table during meals. Whoever has the bell, talking stick, carrot stick, or any other preselected item has the floor and can offer whatever news, joke, or story he or she wants to share. When that person is finished, the bell is passed to the next person. Alternatively, the bell can sit in the middle and whoever wants to say something can take the bell, ring it, and then share.

5. A favorite game in our family, once we finish eating, is to create a story together. One person starts with a word, like "Once," the next person gives a second word, like "there," and it goes on. Hilarious and crazy stories will grow from single words, and it becomes a group effort.

Making Cooking a Family Affair

Here are some simple ideas for fostering connection and mindfulness with your family while you are preparing family meals:

1. Kids are more likely to enjoy eating something they helped to create, so let the children choose a recipe once a week to prepare. Help them make the shopping list, and be sure that you or someone else has the time to assist them in the process. If you are in the kitchen with them, remind them to be in the moment and enjoy the process rather than concentrating on the uncontrollable outcome. Having you there will keep them from feeling frustrated and possibly giving up on the activity entirely. Older children can even develop a specialty, a particular recipe they like to prepare, such as tacos or salads. They can be encouraged to become proficient in various ways to prepare their dish. This also provides the regular cook with a backup on days that are particularly busy.

2. Kids tend to like the same foods over and over, so let the children choose a favorite meal for you to prepare every week or every other week. If you worry too much about giving them the perfect varied diet, you will be focusing only on the outcome; this may begin to generate resentment and it won't be much fun for anyone. The right amount of structure can actually create more spaciousness, so consider allowing one day a week to be "pasta day," one day to be "soup day," and so on, so you don't have to make as many decisions. Too much predictability can become monotonous, so mixing in a brand new meal now and then can keep it fun for everyone.

3. Make carryout food a treat, not a regular activity, and find restaurants that cater to families and that serve healthy food.

4. Take a cooking class with your children.

5. Choose one meal a day, usually dinner, to be a respite from the stress of modern life. One mom told me that her family agreed that they needed some downtime when everyone could be calm and quiet, so they decided together that all electronics in the house would be turned off when it's

time to eat. Alternatively, consider asking the kids to leave electronics in another room during meals.

6. Unless you're a doctor on call or have a pressing emergency, don't bring individual electronics to the table either. If you start from the beginning protecting your dining room table from electronic devices—phones, games, and computers—this situation will be much easier to manage when kids hit the teenage years. Be careful not to open the door to this behavior by bringing your laptop in or letting your teenager text "just this once."

7. When eating with kids, my friend Michelle asks each of her children to say something about what is happening in their mouths. This can be a particular taste, texture, or temperature. Sensing what is happening inside their mouths is a fun way to teach children to eat more mindfully. Like the ban on electronics, rituals like this are best started when the kids are young.

8. Take food-related field trips. If you are a vegetarian or vegan, visit an animal shelter or sanctuary to help the kids understand why you don't eat animal products. One woman I know takes her preteen daughter grocery shopping for a low-income senior. This provides space to talk about how income affects food choices. Pick-your-own farms and cooperative gardens are great for helping children understand how plants are grown and harvested and the impacts of farming.

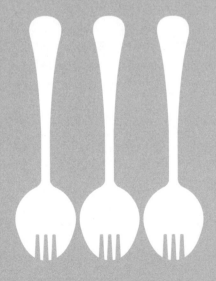

6.

DETAILED INGREDIENTS

*To renounce the sense objects is to torture oneself by asceticism—
don't do it! When you see form, look! Similarly listen to sounds,
inhale scents, taste delicious flavors, feel textures. Use the
objects of the five senses—you will quickly attain Buddhahood.*

—FROM *THE CHANDAMAHAROSANA TANTRA*,
AN EIGHTH-CENTURY BUDDHIST TEXT

It's our third family mindfulness retreat—this one is being held during the late summer at the University of Massachusetts, Amherst. We eat all our mindful meals in the college dining hall, and we sleep together in a single dorm room. This year we know some people from other retreats, and we are starting to feel like we fit in.

As in previous retreats, we spend part of each day in noble silence. Every meal is silent. At our first retreat, there had been a special room for families, because the organizers had recognized how difficult it is for young kids to stay quiet. On this and subsequent retreats, however, there have been no family passes for silence, and we have to try to maintain noble silence alongside everyone else.

Jamie, Lucile, and I are the naturally quiet ones, so it's not as much of a challenge for us. Louie and Veronica, only nine and eleven, like to chatter, so we sometimes pass notes during talks and meals, and when they're noisy I shoot them the if-you-don't-quiet-down-you-will-regret-it-later look. Paul isn't with us; he won't attend a mindfulness retreat for many more years. He's the loudest and most energetic member of our family, and as we are walking silently with the community, Jamie whispers to me rather smugly, "Daddy could never do this."

Because we're on a college campus, the food service is much more standard than when the retreats are held at a Buddhist monastery, where the monks and nuns cook the meals. Instead of bamboo shoots, we get spaghetti. On this day, instead of Vietnamese mung bean soup for dessert, we are treated to blueberry pie.

I am sitting at a round table, trying to eat mindfully along with six hundred other people, when the silence in the hall is suddenly broken. A loud moaning of a child's pleasure is echoing through the hall and getting louder: "Mmmm. Mmmm. MMMMM!…" I feel slightly embarrassed for the child making the noise and even more so for his parents, who will clearly be mortified when they finally hear him. I look toward the sound and am shocked to see my very own Louie, completely immersed in eating his pie. He isn't trying to be loud—he's focused on his pie—he's simply relishing every bite with great joy as if it were the first food he had eaten in months.

SIX HUNDRED PAIRS OF EYES turned toward Louie, some with annoyance, some rolling their eyes, some smiling, and some looking like they wish they could enjoy their food with as much intensity and pleasure as Louie. Seeing him eat with such natural mindfulness and joy inspired me and gave me hope that I might one day rediscover that feeling for myself.

But how? How can we experience the sensory pleasures of food the way we did as children?

As children, most of us are naturally mindful eaters; we only slowly lose our connection to the sense pleasure of our food as we get older. When Marshall Rosenberg described children's joy at feeding ducks and suggested that we only do things that give us that same joy, he was, in essence, suggesting that we reconnect to our senses and experience things the way most of us did as children.

The basic practice of mindful cooking and eating is simply this: In each moment, if your mind wanders away from what you are doing, simply notice that you've been gone. Then, without judgment, return your attention to your physical sensory experience, whether you're smelling the cracked black pepper as it falls onto a fried egg or tasting the fiery flavors of spicy refried pinto beans. Mindfulness in the kitchen is all about our senses. It's that easy.

Sense Food

I love seeing rainbows, but I never fully understood what created them until I read Alan Watts's *The Book: On the Taboo Against Knowing Who You Are.* There he describes how all things rely on each other to manifest: "A rainbow appears only when there is a certain triangular relationship between three components: the sun, moisture in the atmosphere, and an observer. If all three are present, and if the angular relationship between them is correct, then, and then only, will there be the phenomenon 'rainbow.' Diaphanous as it may be, a rainbow is no subjective hallucination. It can be verified by any number of observers, though each will see it in a slightly different position."

A rainbow isn't just an objective reality in the sky; it is created by what is outside of us: the sun and the atmosphere—and also what is inside of us: our human eyes. If we had the eyes of a dog, we would see something very different. What we experience is founded entirely on our five senses and then shaped by our minds.

It turns out that the data that enters our senses gets massaged quite a bit before we "make sense" of it. Our sense organs and our minds rely on each other to create the world as we experience it. It's not unusual for me to think I see someone I know, but when I get closer, I see it's not them. There's a game I use to illustrate this in my children's yoga classes in which I slowly ring a bell five to fifteen times while the students silently listen. When I stop ringing it, they write down how many times they thought it was rung. No matter how carefully we all listen, there is never any consensus about the number of times it sounded. Everyone's mind has added or taken away something from the experience. I can't even be sure that I have the right number because our experiences are so subjective.

If we include the mind as a sense organ, as the Buddhists do, then everything we experience comes to us through one of our sense "doors." We have the five usual sense organs: eyes, ears, nose, tongue, and the body. The sixth sense "door," through which things enter us, is our mind. Once we realize that our whole world is created by these six senses, we are motivated to pay attention to what comes in and to what our mind adds or subtracts.

Our mind is always interpreting external data. Our neighbor Jim regularly comes out to chat with us when he sees us walking into our house. One day recently, when we drove up to our house, Paul and I saw Jim on his front porch as we stepped out of our car. Normally, he would have waved and bellowed something about his day or asked us something about ours. This time, he nodded but didn't say a word.

Paul and I both experienced this encounter and yet our minds concocted completely different stories about it. As we walked up our front steps, I thought, "Oh no, I must have done something to piss off Jim." Paul turned to me and said, "It's so sad, Jim must be depressed." I cracked up. We had the same sensory input, but we interpreted it in completely opposite ways based on our individual and social conditioning, genetics, and experiences. Paul doesn't have a habit of blaming himself like I do, so he assumed that Jim's problem was Jim's alone, and I assumed Jim's actions were a result of something I did wrong. Our minds were trying to make sense of our sensory input.

Practicing mindfulness as we consider what we are taking in through our five senses can help us determine what our mind is adding to every situation. In reality, we can only pay full attention to what our senses are experiencing in this very moment. We can have a memory of a smell, taste, or sound, but when we are actually smelling, tasting, or hearing something, it is happening now. Thoughts and ideas can bring us to other worlds and other times, but our senses bring us back home to this moment—the only moment in which we can actually experience life.

It's impossible to remember making a meal when I didn't get lost in thinking at least once or twice. When I rush through the process of preparing multiple dishes, I often start to lose track of my senses and get caught up in thinking about getting it done, putting it on the table, and sitting down to enjoy it. If I stay present for my senses, I find that it's possible to enjoy and even relax while I'm cooking.

Frequently, someone comes into the kitchen while I'm preparing a meal, and they almost always make a comment like, "Oh, that smells great!" Until that point, I probably have forgotten to notice the smells myself! Trying to stay present in the kitchen is just like trying to stay present in meditation. As soon as I notice that my mind is dashing off into the future (getting the meal onto the table) or lingering and obsessing about the past (rehashing a stressful conversation), I invite my mind back into the moment by feeling the coolness of the rice water, noticing the deep burgundy color of the freshly peeled beets, or breathing in the aroma of the sautéed onions.

Our senses are the doorways into the experience of our life. No idea or thought can compare to the joy of seeing my daughter's smiling face again after she came out of a harrowing abdominal surgery or hearing my teenage son's voice on the phone while he was living in France. And while our senses very often bring us pain as well, staying present for them helps prevent us from shooting the second arrow; we learn to tolerate our feelings rather than run away from them. Like the proverbial monster under the bed, our sense experiences are less scary when we face them directly.

On Sight

When I was eleven, my family and I traveled to Ecuador to pick up my sister Maggie from her year abroad in Quito. We added a side trip to Machu Picchu in Peru and returned home by way of Cuzco. It was my first trip out of the country, my first time at such an altitude, and also the first time I ate plantains. I didn't have to worry about eating too much on this trip, because there wasn't too much that I enjoyed, so by the time we found the lightly browned and buttery plantains sold by a street vendor, I went a little crazy. I ate dozens of them.

I noticed that I didn't feel very well the next morning, and by the time we boarded our flight back to the US, I was throwing up. When we landed in Panama to refuel (this was 1973), the humidity was nearly one hundred percent and it must have been ninety-eight degrees. The paper bag was my best friend for the next leg of the flight home.

I got over my plantain revulsion some years later when I ordered them at our favorite Mexican restaurant and I realized that I did indeed love them. I hadn't considered making them myself because I was unfamiliar with how they were prepared—I had never seen them cooked or served at anyone's home. But one day last year, I thought, "What the hell," and bought a few at the local market. They were the color of ripe bananas but they didn't have any smell at all. And they were probably hard enough to pound nails.

I heated up some canola oil and tried to cut the rigid plantains into pieces. No luck. I pulled out the largest cleaver I had and went at them. Eventually I managed to chunk them up and I tossed the rock-hard chunks into the oil. They browned nicely, but they didn't soften at all. I don't really know why I served them—I guess I thought they looked pretty. Everyone hated them, including me. Not only were they nearly impossible to chew, but they tasted like banana peel.

The next day, a day too late, I Googled "how to cook plantains" and learned that plantains need to look like rotten bananas before they are ready to cook. So the next time I bought them, I let them lounge on the kitchen counter for two weeks until they looked terrible. They were mostly black, rotten-looking, and quite squishy, but they finally smelled ripe. I fried them up and voilà, delicious plantains! I needed to know how to see and smell ripe plantains before I could make them taste delicious.

Experimenting with food uses all of our senses. If our eyesight is good, the sense we'll probably rely on most is our sight. We can learn a lot about food by simply looking at the ingredients we are cooking with or the dish we are about to eat. What color is it? Is it all one color? If so, are there gradations in that color? Is it glossy or matte? Does it have an odd or interesting shape? If it turns brown when it cooks, is it a deep, dark brown or a luminescent tan? Does it have brown blotches, or is it one consistent shade? All of these are clues to working effectively with food and learning what needs to happen next.

A friend of mine describes the experience of looking at ingredients and finished food as "going to an art museum." A single cabbage leaf can provide a world of beauty and joy if we take the time to study its shape and how it is put together. Some cabbages are purple, some are green, and some are closer to white. Some have soft crinkled leaves, and some are tight and flat. If we look at the whole cabbage, we might notice it resembles a rose with petal after petal radiating out from the central core. Who knew you could spend so much time admiring a head of cabbage?

What's more, our food—unlike the images we're used to seeing on our TV or computer screens—is three-dimensional, it's real. It even has a culture. Consider, again, the cabbage. According to Wikipedia, Egyptian pharaohs believed that if they ate enough cabbage while drinking, they wouldn't have a hangover. Captain Cook apparently used cabbage leaves on his ship as bandages, and many people in the southern US and parts of Europe and

Asia eat cabbage on New Year's Eve for good luck. Many of our foods have a long, fascinating history that we can learn and think about when we are cooking.

In the US a growing number of people are interested in knowing something about where their food came from and how it was handled before it reached their plate. Every meal has a long history, some of which we can know and some of which we can only guess at. If we know, for example, the organic farmer who grows our vegetables, we will be happy to eat her food because it makes us feel good to support her livelihood. If we find out that her farmworkers are not paid a fair wage and that they can't afford to eat the vegetables they grow, we might not enjoy them as much. Until recently, most of us ate our food without awareness of its origins. As author Wendell Berry reminds us, "A significant part of the pleasure of eating is in one's accurate consciousness of the lives and the world from which the food comes."

On Sound

When was the last time you listened to your food? Most food is silent once it hits the table (with the exception of flaming Greek saganaki cheese or sizzling Mexican fajitas), but many foods make noise while they are cooking. When vegetables steam, rice boils, or the pressure cooker cools, you can hear it.

I like to listen to the sounds of the kitchen, because they bring me back to my senses and tell me what is happening with my food. When I hear the water boiling, I know it's time to add the pasta; when I hear the soy butter start to sizzle, I know it's time to add the onions. It's likely that kitchen sounds aren't the only things you hear when you're cooking. On a typical day in my kitchen, I hear the garbage trucks rolling through the alley, dogs barking, doors slamming, someone taking a shower, and a car alarm going off—not to mention the sounds coming from inside my own head.

Recent studies on food and sounds show that listening to high-pitched sounds causes people to taste sweetness, while listening to lower-pitched music causes them to taste bitterness. Loud background music, like the noise of flying on a plane, reduces our ability to taste anything at all, which could partially explain why airplane food can taste so awful.

Sounds, on their own, aren't good or bad—they are simply sound waves landing on our eardrums. Some sounds, like classical music or waves on the shore, tend to be relaxing for most people, whereas other sounds, like my little dogs yipping at every person who walks by the house, usually create stress. I once heard Ram Dass suggest that in the right state of mind, we can even use the sound of an ambulance as "free energy from the universe." When we simply hear a sound, without resistance, it can inspire us with its vitality rather than create more tension.

Find your own way to use sound to bring you back to the moment. You may want to create a quiet zone in the kitchen so you can hear your food more clearly. If you don't have that luxury—if you have children, dogs, or a noisy environment—then you might just need to practice, like Ram Dass, using the sounds in your environment as energy for your mindful cooking.

On Smell

Sometimes when I'm out walking the dogs on a Saturday morning, I get a waft of bacon from a neighbor's kitchen, and I am immediately transported back in time. Our oldest child, Lucile, was a huge bacon fan, and most weekends we went through at least one whole package of the stuff. When I think of that, a huge smile breaks out on my face. Smell is like that.

Smells and tastes are actually more likely to bring back memories than hearing words or seeing images. This reaction is often referred to as the "Proust Effect," based on the novelist's famous description, in *Swann's Way*, of tasting a madeleine cookie and suddenly remembering his Aunt Leonie giving him a madeleine as a child. He wrote, "But when from a long-distant past nothing subsists, after the people are dead, after the things are broken and scattered, taste and smell alone, more fragile but more enduring, more unsubstantial, more persistent, more faithful, remain poised a long time, like souls, remembering, waiting, hoping, amid the ruins of all the rest; and bear unflinchingly, in the tiny and almost impalpable drop of their essence, the vast structure of recollection."[7]

Proust's sudden memory brings him "an exquisite pleasure," an "all-powerful joy." We can use our own underused sense of smell to create more joy in our kitchen. Everything we cook has distinctive smells, and learning to rely on your olfactory sense can help you cook delicious food more easily and create long-lasting pleasant memories for yourself, your friends, and family.

Smell every ingredient before you use it. Notice the subtle differences between the smell of a baking russet potato and a sweet potato. Compare the smell of a strawberry grown locally to one grown thousands of miles away. Notice the smell of whole grains getting sweeter as they cook. As you crack open the pepper with the pepper mill, savor the essence of the pepper as it is released into the atmosphere where your nose receives it. With enough practice, you may be able to tell when something is done cooking without lifting the lid or opening the oven.

Your sense of smell also plays a big role in your ability to taste. The olfactory receptors in our noses, along with the receptors in our mouths, are what define the taste of our food before we even begin eating, and it doesn't end when we start to eat. As we chew, more smell is released into our nose, which increases our ability to taste. Before eating, inhale deeply the smell of your food. Then, as you continue your meal, pause now and then to smell again, and see how your sense of smell continues to enrich your experience.

On Taste

Many times when my kids were young, I prepared and ate my dinner standing up while serving them at the table, all the while thinking about the million and one things I had to do that night: answer questions from staff and students about the studio, prepare to teach a class, make sure the kids' homework was done, and return phone calls. Only afterward, while washing the dishes, would I ask myself, "What did I just eat? What did it taste like?" I missed the flavor of many of the meals with my children. Though we may never achieve full-time mindfulness, we can start to enjoy more of these moments, whether eating alone or with loved ones, through the portal of taste.

Tasting food is the most obvious way to practice mindfulness when cooking and eating. Of course we taste everything when we eat, right? And yet, how many times have you finished eating something and wondered where it went? You didn't even notice you were eating it.

Tasting food can also be an antidote to emotional eating. The more I taste my food, the more I am present, because I am not numbing out. If we don't taste the food we are eating, we'll want more when our plate is empty because our minds haven't registered that we ate. It's as if we haven't really eaten anything at all.

If we miss the taste of an apple while eating it, then we miss the enjoyment of that apple, and all the efforts of the tree, the sun, the rain, and the farmer are lost. Slowing down to truly taste our food is a way of respecting all of the people, animals, plants, and minerals that went into our meal. It also helps stop us eating out of habit, so we are less likely to overeat or binge.

Scientists believe we have five different types of taste buds on our tongues: receptors for sweet, bitter, sour, salty, and *unami* (savory) flavors. In the last decade, cellular biologists have discovered that we also have taste buds in many other places, including our stomach, intestines, and pancreas. These non-mouth taste buds help us digest our food by influencing our appetite and regulating insulin. Research is still underway on why we have taste buds in places like our airways and—yes, really—in sperm.[8]

But be warned, taste buds can be fooled. One year, Paul got interested in the West African "miracle fruit" (a.k.a. *Synsepalum dulcificum*) that, when eaten, causes any sour food eaten afterward to taste sweet. Apparently, the miracle berry leaves a residue of protein in our mouths that activates the sweet-taste receptors whenever it comes into contact with a low pH (sour) food. He ordered several bags of the frozen berries, and in lieu of dinner one evening, we had a Miracle Fruit Party with our kids and a bunch of their friends. We filled the dining room table with plates of the sourest foods we could find—lemon and lime wedges, vinegar, pickles, and sour cream—and then we each chewed up a berry or two.

After swallowing the berries, I chomped right into a huge lemon wedge and was astounded to discover that it was now sweet lemonade. We poured and drank whole glasses of apple cider vinegar, which tasted like sweet apple cider, and then we ate sour cream that reminded us of cheesecake. After about twenty minutes, the effect wore off and sour foods became sour again.

Of course, you can use your taste buds while cooking too. As the cook, taste is how you communicate to your diners. When I taste the parsnip soup I am making, I decide what other ingredients or seasoning it needs based on what I want my friends and family to taste when I serve it. I'm passing a nonverbal message from my mouth to theirs. If my taste buds say a dish needs more salt, my diners get more salt. If they say spicy, they get spicy.

Like all the other senses, taste offers us a direct route to the present moment. When we taste our food, we slow down the process of eating by bringing it into our body instead of only our minds. We are really eating food, not just thinking about eating food. The more I have been able to taste my food, the less I feel the need to binge. The more I learn what food tastes like, the easier cooking becomes, because I know what I like and what tastes good. As Homer wisely says in the Simpsons episode, "The Food Wife": "I don't want to think about food, I want to like it."

On Touch

When Veronica was young, she always wanted to be touching us. When we walked to school she would yell, "Carry my hand, mama, carry my hand!" On a cold winter morning, sometimes my meditation starts with being aware of my husband lying in my arms next to me, or the soft warm covers and the weight of my two small terriers hogging the bed. I call this "beditation."

I remember how natural it felt to eat with my hands before I learned that it wasn't acceptable to touch our food. A Laotian restaurant near my house serves individual baskets of warm, slightly sweet, sticky rice; when we eat there, I get to open the baskets, take a small clump into my hand, dip it in sauce, and eat. It's one of the few places where it's still acceptable to eat with my hands, and I love it!

Our hands, however, aren't the only part of our body that feels things. We feel on the outside with our skin and some mucosa, and also on the inside (temperature, balance, our perception of where our body is in space, pain, and the like). Think about the difference between the feeling of eating warm rice pudding and of eating a cold, crisp apple. We keep "touching" our food until it gets into our stomach.

On one silent meditation retreat, I began to notice the feeling of the food making its way down my esophagus. It was a strange sensation, but I was able to track my food from the time it arrived in my mouth until it landed in my stomach. Keeping my attention trained in this way slowed down the process. I ate only what my body really wanted and enjoyed each bite thoroughly. It wasn't a sustainable practice once I left the retreat—I just didn't have the patience to eat that slowly at home. But it did raise my awareness enough so that from time to time I remember to feel my food until it gets to my stomach.

We tend to underutilize our sense of touch in cooking. Bringing our attention to the bumpy surface of a kale leaf, the warmth coming from our oven, the roughness of the rice kernels as we wash them, or the gelatinous texture of chia pudding as it sets can be fun and always brings us back to the present moment.

In addition to smell and taste, our sense of touch can add another dimension of wisdom to our cooking. We can train ourselves to know something is ready to eat simply by touching it—the ripeness of a piece of fruit, the thickness of a soup, or the doneness of a potato.

On Mind

On nights when my mind is hijacked by my habitual thoughts, I'm not able to experience any of my other senses. This is a regular occurrence. I start to cook, and I'm seeing the color of the lettuce leaves, smelling the olive oil, onions, and garlic as I mix up a dressing, hearing the artist Phamie Gow's piano music playing through a speaker. And then I get lost. I'm thinking about something I'm writing, or my daughter's newest relationship, or the fact that tomorrow is my wedding anniversary and I don't even have a card for my sweet husband. From there, my mind goes into planning mode—I'll write this, or I'll tell my daughter that, or maybe I have a blank card in the drawer that I can use. My mind goes off for a couple of minutes or more while I am chopping, mixing, and stirring. I'm just not there.

I've learned from mindfulness practice that this is normal. And because it's normal, there is no use in getting upset about it. It happens. I attended a retreat once with the venerable Buddhist nun Pema Chödrön, in which she said, "After all these years of meditation, I just accept that I have a very busy mind." If a Buddhist nun who has been meditating consistently for over forty years still has a busy mind, I know I'm in good company.

When our minds are off ruminating God-knows-where, time seems to fly by. Suddenly the plate is empty, dinner is over, summer has passed, and we've missed it. The practice of mindfulness may give us the feeling that we have slowed time and have more of it. Neuroscientist David Eagleman, author of *Incognito: The Secret Lives of The Brain*, has studied how attention to something novel makes us feel that time is slowing down (he calls this the "oddball effect").[9]

In one of his studies, he presents subjects with sounds or pictures that are mostly repetitive and occur at regular intervals. When subjects are presented with a unique sound or picture, it seems, to them, that the unusual sound or picture is on the screen for a longer duration. It isn't. It's just how our minds process new information.

That means that we can expand time right in our own homes by notic-ing what is new and pleasant—whether it's the color of a ripe peach, the sound of popcorn, or your first bite of fresh homemade applesauce. "Time is this rubbery thing," Eagleman says. "It stretches out when you really turn your brain resources on, and when you say, 'Oh, I got this, everything is as expected,' it shrinks up." So, practicing mindfulness may be just what you need if you feel that you don't have enough time to be mindful!

Although we can explore each of our senses separately, in reality our senses are always working together. We rarely taste or smell something without having looked at it first, and our ears, when they are working, are always turned on. When we bite into a piece of cinnamon toast, for example, we see the golden brown-speckled loaf shape, hear the dramatic crunching, experience the peppery sweet buttery aroma, sense the mixture of dry and moist sensation inside our mouths (and the slick feeling on our lips), and quite possibly have a mental image, memory, or thought, before our taste buds even get involved. All six senses combine to create what we call the "taste" or "flavor" of our food. When we are really in the zone of our senses, we can taste not just the flavor of our food, but the full flavor of our lives.

The Middle Way

Think about the moment you step into a warm shower after a long day of working, after a run, a sweaty yoga class, or digging in the garden. Then think about being forced to stay in the same hot shower for two hundred days, which is how many hours we spend, on average, showering in our lifetimes. Not so pleasant, is it? Or think about your favorite food. Now imagine that you have to eat that food three times a day for the next twenty-five years. It doesn't sound as tasty, does it? That's because joy doesn't stem from our senses alone. Joy actually also rests on the insight of impermanence—the constantly changing nature of life.

Most of us think that if a little of something is good, a lot must be better. But too much of a good thing dulls our ability to enjoy it. Unfortunately, our minds forget this, which is why our senses can actually increase our suffering if we don't remember the Buddha's teaching of "the Middle Way."

The person who we call the Buddha was born Siddhartha Gautama, a prince in ancient India. According to the Buddhist texts, Siddhartha enjoyed a privileged lifestyle with access to great food, drink, clothing, and music. When he left home as a young man, he became an ascetic—someone who renounced sensual pleasures. For Siddhartha, this meant that he wore very little, slept on the ground, and lived on one single grain of rice each day. As a result, he became extremely thin and quite sick.

Trying to live without any sensual pleasures is neither pleasant nor is it a relief from suffering. Siddhartha was dying of hunger and thirst when he realized that his asceticism wasn't bringing him closer to answering the question he had set out to answer: how to reduce human suffering. He was overwrought and in pain, his eyes sunken into their sockets, his ribs jutting out, and his scalp shriveled and withered "as a green bitter gourd shrivels and withers in the wind and sun." He was no closer to freeing himself or the world from suffering.

As he lay dying, Siddhartha remembered a wonderful moment when as a child he had sat quietly under the cool shade of a rose-apple tree. He knew already that indulgence was not the way, but now he realized that asceticism was not the way either, and that he needed to eat if he was going to be able to reach enlightenment. So he began to take nourishment again.[10]

As a result of this experience, the Buddha told his students not to go to either extreme—not bingeing on sensual pleasure nor denying themselves pleasurable sensations. Emotional eating, bingeing, skipping meals, and purging are painful ways we live out these extremes. When we eat mindlessly, we are craving the sensual pleasures of food and we believe that if we eat, we will be truly and completely happy. When we deny ourselves food, we do the opposite. More than two thousand years after the Buddha taught the Middle Way, it remains relevant because many of us still live in one extreme or another.[11]

He goes on to say that happiness, not the transitory exciting kind but the long-lasting contentment kind, is maximized by enjoying ourselves—tasting and smelling our food, listening to lovely music, looking at beautiful scenes—but not to the point of clinging, obsessing, or over-indulging. If we ate tiramisu for three meals a day, we wouldn't enjoy it very much after a while. But when we eat a bite of it once on occasion, it's simply wonderful.

Cooking as Meditation

When I was a child, I would sometimes stay overnight at my grandma's house. After an evening spent watching the movie *Heidi* curled up together in her La-Z-Boy, she tucked me in and sang me to sleep with the song, "Let's Go a Huntin'." I woke the next morning in the small bedroom that my mom had slept in while growing up, and I slid down the old oak banister to wake up Grandma.

The house was usually chilly, so I wore the quilted pink robe my grandma had made me over my pajamas. I always had a single soft-boiled egg and one piece of toasted homemade bread for breakfast, all of it prepared and eaten mindfully. Grandma let me pick out an egg from the egg carton and watch her boil it on the stove. There was an hourglass timer to let us know when the egg would be ready, and during those few minutes, we would choose my egg cup from the many curious ones in her cupboard. The pink cup shaped like a pig's face was my favorite.

When the egg had finished cooking, Grandma carefully lifted it out of the water with a slotted spoon and rinsed it momentarily under cool water before placing it in my cup. Then we took the chicken-shaped egg chopper off the wall where it always hung, and waited for the egg to cool enough to break it open. While the egg was cooling, we cut and toasted a piece of her homemade bread. When it popped out of the toaster, Grandma let me spread the butter before she cut it diagonally. By then, the egg was ready to be broken open with the egg chopper.

Cooking with Grandma was a kind of meditation. One simple egg was all it took; by the time I sat down to eat, I was completely present with my food.

Size Doesn't Matter

The old Michigan farmhouse where I grew up originally had teeny-tiny bedrooms and a huge kitchen and pantry. When the house was built in 1835, the kitchen was the heart of the house, where the family came together to cook, eat, and connect. In American farmhouses like ours, kitchens were grand communal spaces.

When I was still a baby, my parents renovated the house and broke the kitchen up into different rooms. Designed for efficiency, not enjoyment, our new kitchen was barely big enough to hold two people. Our renovation reflected a similar shift in thinking about home cooking and meals that was taking place all over the US in the 1970s and 1980s. Many more families than in the past had two working parents, and cooking was becoming more utilitarian—it was one more job to do before or after a hard day at work.

Between 1965 and the late 1990s, Americans' consumption of home-cooked food decreased, along with time spent cooking. A 2011 survey by LivingSocial found that in the US the average adult eats five meals per week outside the home.[12] A 2013 study from *Nutritional Journal* reported that only a bit more than half of Americans spend any time at all cooking on a given day.[13] While Laurie David, cookbook author and producer of the film *Fed Up*, a documentary exploring the causes of obesity in the US, says, "Not to cook in your own home is to miss one of the best parts of the day," a lot of us simply don't have the time or inclination to cook after a hard day at work or a long commute.

If working and commuting doesn't cut into time spent cooking, taking care of a family will. As parents spend more time than ever driving kids to school, sports, and other activities, it gets harder and harder to find the time to cook, let alone cook mindfully. Nearly ten percent of Americans surveyed in a US Energy Information Administration survey in 2009 said that they make most, if not all, of their meals and snacks in the microwave.[14]

Eating out doesn't necessarily mean we aren't eating mindfully, but it does disconnect us more from the elements of a meal than cooking at home does, and from the process of preparing food for ourselves or our friends and family. The idea and practice of cooking as an enjoyable and meditative practice has been lost for many of us. Even if we can find the time to cook, we may think we aren't capable because we didn't learn the art from our parents.

Meanwhile, our country is experiencing an explosion in foodie culture, which can be unnecessarily confusing and intimidating to novice cooks. If you don't know whether you are a locavore, vegan, lacto-ovo, fruitarian, raw food fan, vegetarian, or omnivore—if you don't have a clue what to do with arugula and daikon radishes, or you don't watch Iron Chef—it's okay! You don't need to know anything special to cook and enjoy simple meals mindfully and to experience food with all your senses. Sometimes, all you need is a simple egg and your mindful presence.

As Laurie David suggests, "The single healthiest activity you can do with your family is cook and eat meals together. Discover the joy in the process; put music on, light a candle, have everyone participate. Then it's not all on you, and everyone's going to have fun doing it. You can't cut a carrot with one hand and text with the other! Everyone needs a break from technology. What a perfect way to take that break—by making dinner and sitting down to enjoy it."

Cooking as meditation doesn't require a spacious kitchen or a lot of time. In the beginning, it's helpful to set aside a few extra minutes to pause and bring yourself back to your senses when you start to ruminate about projects or problems. If you cook when you are already hungry, it might be difficult to stay present, so if possible, cook when you aren't desperately hungry, or else have a nutritious snack, like crackers and hummus, before you start.

Your Kitchen, Your Temple

No matter what's happening in my life, I can always go into the kitchen and work with it. If I'm happy, I can cook. If I'm angry or sad, I can still cook. My kitchen is like my meditation cushion, so I try to create an environment that supports my practice of mindful cooking.

I have a shelf where I put small reminders—a kind of kitchen altar. Right now it has a picture of my mother and my maternal grandmother, the women who fed me and taught me how to cook. There's also a female Buddha statue on the shelf, two calligraphies that I wrote—one says "Joy" and the other says "Eat to Live," a felt flower made by a friend, an origami peace swan given to me by a young student, and a postcard of a photograph of a little boy running with a baguette. My husband gave it to me with a note that said, "You are the baguette I run with, and we smile and run together." All these items remind me of my purpose in the kitchen: to be present for the nourishment I am creating for myself and others, to enjoy the whole amazing process, and to have fun!

Another way that I support my practice of mindful cooking, eating, and connecting to my senses is to post reminders that bring me back to the present moment. If you visit my kitchen, you'll see pieces of paper taped to the walls and cabinets. One says, "You can search the whole world over but you will never find anyone more deserving of your love and care than you yourself." Near the garbage it says,

In the garbage, I see a rose.
In the rose, I see compost.
Everything is in transformation.
Impermanence is life.

I bought a piece of calligraphy on my first mindfulness retreat that said "Breathe, my dear." It has been hanging in my kitchen for more than a decade. These signs remind me to come back to my breathing and consider the interbeing and impermanence of life, and also to be gentle with my practice and myself. (See the "Kitchen Gathas" on page 178 for more ideas on kitchen mindfulness notes.)

I also keep a copy of The Five Contemplations (see Appendices page 236) on my kitchen table. The Five Contemplations are verses reminding us of all the conditions that have come together to make this meal possible. Similar contemplations have been recited in meditation centers around the world using different words to express the same reminders:

1. Remembering everyone and everything that had a hand in bringing the food to us;
2. Reminding ourselves to be grateful for this food;
3. Reminding ourselves of the human habit of always wanting more, and becoming aware that we don't have to act from that craving while we eat this meal and we can eat with moderation;
4. Remembering that the purpose of eating this food is for our own health;
5. Remembering our life's intention, which is being kept alive by the food on our plates.

Before eating alone I often recite the contemplations to myself; when eating with the mindfulness Sangha, we recite them together. Sometimes we read them at home, especially if we have guests who are expecting grace. When I first heard them, I was so excited that I read them aloud at Thanksgiving dinner with my extended family at my cousin's house. When I finished reading, everyone looked around the table awkwardly. Had I just proposed moderation during a Thanksgiving feast?

Consider how you might create a mindful kitchen environment for yourself. Play your favorite music while you cook, set up a kitchen altar, leave little love notes for yourself, post reminders to be mindful or favorite mindfulness quotes, clear out clutter, or rearrange the furniture. Use your creativity and imagination to make your cooking and eating space a haven for mindfulness and nourishment for yourself and anyone who enters.

I just posted this note by an unknown author: "Peace. It does not mean to be in a place where there is no noise, trouble, or hard work. It means to be in the midst of those things and still be calm in your heart." You may not want to plaster your walls with sticky notes like I do, but find your own way to remind yourself to keep coming back to your senses and find peace.

Going Solo

When my aunt Nancy got divorced, she made a decision not to punish herself for being single by eating meals that were thoughtless, on the run, unhealthy, or uninteresting. She decided that if she cared enough about other people to cook well for them—like she did for her son, for example— then she could do the same for herself. Even when she is alone, she cooks a nice meal, sets the table, turns on her favorite music, and enjoys herself. She builds a fire for herself in the winter, and in warmer months, she eats on her porch in her grandfather's rocker. Her motto is, "Why not take care of yourself as well as you take care of others?"

It might feel awkward to be alone in silence, and difficult not to be distracted by the talking, planning, and ruminating in your own mind. It's tempting for all of us to read a book or surf the web while eating. When we prepare or eat meals alone and are fully present for our food, it's possible that unpleasant emotions like anger or fear might show up, but we don't have to run away from those feelings. Instead, sit down with your restlessness or your fear. Let it be there beside you. Get to know it. "Hello, awkwardness." "Hello, fear." Even with the awkwardness there, you can still stay present for your meal. Then the awkwardness is no longer in charge—you are.

Even after years of mindfulness practice, I still feel awkward when I eat alone with no distractions. But now I know how to say hello to that awkwardness. For me, what underlies the discomfort is a feeling of urgency, as though I shouldn't be wasting my time eating. Paying attention to my senses and allowing myself to linger over the tastes and smells of food feels selfish. There are better, more important things and people who need my attention, and I should get going! If I apply the Middle Way to my thoughts, I see that while indulging myself in a sensual binge isn't a route to happiness, neither is abstaining from enjoying a delectable meal.

And let's just be honest. There are plenty of times that I do read or Google while I am eating just because I want to. But when I decide to do that, I don't judge or condemn myself. I just do it. The part of me that wants to be distracted is here too. All of it is welcome.

When I sit down to eat alone, I always begin with a moment of gratitude. Sometimes I say the Five Contemplations, but sometimes I just smile and bow to my food. I acknowledge that a lot of beings have made it possible for me to eat this food and be nourished. Sometimes I set my intention to use the nourishment I am receiving for the benefit of my community or my family.

When I finish eating, I look at my empty plate and remember what it looked like when it was full. I remind myself that all that food is now inside me. And I wonder, what will I do with that energy?

The Zen Master Katagiri Roshi once said, "When eating, just eat. When reading, just read. When eating and reading, just eat and read." The same applies to your awkwardness while eating alone. "When eating and feeling awkward, just eat and feel awkward." No big deal. Whatever you are doing, the practice is to bring your full attention to what is happening. Our senses are what bring us back to the present moment—tasting, smelling, listening, touching, and seeing what is on our plate. By paying attention to our senses, we will be able to truly be here with whatever arises.

Mind the Gaps

Remember that our minds have the ability to fill in gaps in our sense experiences; the mind will naturally combine and magnify information we gather through our senses. We might not always be aware of the misperceptions we produced based on what we hear or see. We hear someone walking up the sidewalk toward our house, for example, and we imagine it's a magazine salesman and we get annoyed. But when we look outside, it's our Chinese food delivery! It could have been the neighbor's dog or the melting ice, but our mind creates an entire story and a reaction based on a few sounds. Our mind fills in the gaps.

If we don't see the way that our mind is working in the background, we will continue to live in a delusion. If we really want to wake up, we have to remember that our mind is always trying to make sense of our senses. We taste food and know that our taste buds are simply touching a substance in our mouths. Our mind tells us that it's delicious and that eating it will solve all our problems! We know it's just a taste-bud effect and a pleasurable sensation, not a panacea for all of our problems, so we can choose to take another bite or not. We can enjoy every minute of our sense experience without holding it too tightly. We can choose the Middle Way.

The Buddha said, "This is because that is." What you prepare and what you eat have an effect that radiates out. What you put into your body becomes who you are and what you bring to the world. In the 1960s, the slogan "You are what you eat" was everywhere. On a molecular level, we really are made up of all the food that we eat. But we are so much more.

In recent years countless films have been made and many books published on the realities of factory farming, agribusiness, and food security. But our physical and mental health also depends on what we take in through our lungs, our skin, and our minds. The Buddha suggested that what we consume can be divided into four categories: edible food, sense impressions, volition (what we desire), and consciousness (what we think and what our society thinks). (See the Four Nutriments on page 172.)

We're All Doing Time

I teach mindfulness in a women's jail twice a month. It's an environment in which mindfulness is vital and yet difficult to sow. Besides the usual challenges, most of the women have told us that they feel lethargic and heavy; some have gained twenty to fifty pounds while incarcerated (which in this facility is usually not more than one year). They tell me the meals there are carbohydrate- and salt-heavy and that they get very little exercise.

Most of the women are depressed because they are separated from their loved ones. I would guess that their depression is made worse by their unhealthy diets and they overeat because they are depressed. It seems that jail must be one of the hardest places to be mindful. And yet mindfulness is possible no matter what our circumstances.

In an article in *Shambhala Sun* magazine, correctional prisoner Scott Darnell describes how he worked with an extremely difficult moment in prison: "I thought about how I had an obligation to live what I had earned as fully as I could. At the moment, it happened to be rather difficult. So I decided to sit with the difficulty, opening myself as fully as possible to my situation, whether that was the numbness growing in my fingers due to the cuffs, or the almost jovial banter of the officers as they picked several inmates out of the crowd for a strip search, or the groans, coughs, and covert attempts at shifting positions that everyone was making around me… what I could do was face this moment with them, exercising clarity, awareness, and compassion."[15]

Death Row inmate Jarvis Jay Masters describes in this same article how meditation and mindfulness have changed his life in San Quentin, California's oldest correctional facility and one of the harshest prison environments in the country. "Meditation has become something I cannot do without. I see and hear more clearly, feel more relaxed and calm, and I actually find my experiences slowing down. I'm more appreciative of each day as I observe how things constantly change and dissolve. I've realized that everything is in a continual process of coming and going. I don't hold happiness or anger for a long time. It just comes and goes."

Each of us has our own unique challenges that prevent us from staying in the moment, but our senses are always available to help bring us back to this present. Dropping fully into the sights, smells, and sounds of the moment brings us home to our bodies and to our lives. However, our five senses alone can't bring the end to our suffering. We need to train ourselves to see what is really going on and learn to resist adding the second arrow of suffering to our experiences. Rather than judging ourselves for wanting (or eating) an entire box of cookies, we can notice how we feel instead: "Wanting to eat the entire box of cookies feels like this," or "Having eaten an entire box of cookies feels like this." In this way, we begin to make peace with ourselves and create space for transformation.

Bo Lozoff wrote the landmark book *We're All Doing Time*, published in 1985, which has inspired thousands of prisoners to use meditation and yoga to help transform their experience on the inside. He wrote, "Nothing we ever get, see, taste, smell, touch, hear, or think about is going to bring us the peace we really seek. What clearer reminder do we need that if we're not at peace with ourselves, then we're all doing time in one kind of prison or another? The whole 'spiritual path' is nothing more than being a simple realist about how life works; how the universe operates. We'll always be walking around in maya (illusion), but the trick is to remember that and to honor the rules of the game."

This sentiment is true even if we are physically free. No matter how difficult the moment is, we can survive it and even thrive in it if we learn to become aware of what our conditioned mind might be adding to the moment. As long as we can see and sense the moment as it is, we won't have to struggle with it as much. Learning to pay attention to my senses in the kitchen was like letting go of the rope in the tug-of-war I was having with my eating. Just being there with the smells, sounds, and tastes became enough. Knowing the truth of our senses doesn't mean we won't feel things—it means we can experience life as it is without getting stuck in endless thinking about it, while our brief lives slip by.

This is truly coming to our senses.

||||||||||||||||||||||||||||||||||||||||||||||||||||||||||||||||||||||||||||||||||||||||||||||||||||||

The Four Nutriments

Nutriments are what we take in through our senses that create and shape our lives. Our minds formulate our speech and actions, and our actions lay down neural pathways in our brains, which then become habits. Our bodies and brains have an impact on how we experience the world, which then shapes how we think. The mind and our experiences shape each other. Body and mind are often referred to as the body-mind; they are inseparable. This quote, from the ancient Hindu text, the *Upanishads* describes how the mind can create our world: "Watch your thoughts; they become words. Watch your words; they become actions. Watch your actions; they become habits. Watch your habits; they become character. Watch your character; for it becomes your destiny."

The Buddha taught that there are four nutriments we take into our body and mind. The first nutriment is *edible food*, what we take in through our mouth.

The second nutriment is *sense impressions*, what we take in through our eyes, ears, nose, mouth, body, and mind. Consider the nutriments that you take in through these many doors. Consider all that you have looked at, smelled, listened to, touched, or thought about today. These nutriments are just as important as what we take in through our mouths in the way of food.

My husband and I went to see the movie *A Simple Plan* a few days after I returned from one of my mindfulness retreats. Billy Bob Thornton, his brother, and a friend stumble upon a private plane wreck in the Minnesota woods in which they find over four million dollars in cash. At first they agree that they should share the money and not tell anyone. The movie isn't particularly graphic, but when the brothers begin to secretly turn on each other as a result of their growing greed, my heart, more vulnerable as a result of the retreat, began to ache. By the time one brother had shot the other, I was sobbing uncontrollably and had to leave the theater to the dismay of my husband, who wanted to see the ending.

Choosing what to take in through our senses is a personal matter that changes based on the moment and the situation. On another day, I might have been intellectually stimulated by or simply enjoyed *A Simple Plan*. Watching or reading the news is similar; I keep up with current events, but I try to choose not to overload myself on the violence and misery happening in so much of the world. I know I've overdone it when I fall into despair. When asked what is the most difficult obstacle to the practice of mindfulness, Thich Nhat Hanh answered with one word: "despair." The way to moderate our despair is by choosing our four nutriments carefully.

When I feel overwhelmed, I try to bring something pleasant to my senses. For me, that means taking a walk in nature or in the city. I like being in the woods or on a mountain alone, hearing the wind and the birds, but I also like watching people scurry around a city amidst the colors and shapes of man-made buildings.

I don't bury my head in the sand, but I'm very careful about what I see on the Internet or TV. I now choose to learn mainly about suffering that is real (no need to take in extra suffering in violent movies or books), and that has the potential to awaken compassion in me. Find your own ways to reboot when you've overdone challenging sense inputs: Determine for yourself what sense inputs most support your ability to stay present and at ease, and try to minimize those that keep you distracted or miserable.

Volition, the third of the four nutriments, describes our intentions or our deepest desires and beliefs. What is it that we most want from life? What would you do if you weren't afraid to do it? What do you love most? Our deepest desires affect us even when we aren't conscious of them. If you look into your heart, you will find that there are some underlying desires that may be subtly directing your life.

I believe that if any one of us looks deeply enough, we will find that our deepest aspirations, once we have met our basic needs for living, are to love and be loved, to inspire and serve others, to have fun, to be authentic, and to feel a sense of belonging to a community. Many of us also probably have other desires that we aren't aware of that may not point us in a helpful direction. It could be that we desire to prove ourselves as competent, that we have the need to always be right, or that we want to be powerful and in control.

Our lives are directed by our volitions—those that lead to more ease, but also those that cause us (or our loved ones) to suffer. Becoming more mindful includes becoming aware of how we are driven by our unconscious desires. When we are more conscious of our volitions, we have new awareness of the desires that don't serve us well and new options for minimizing their strength and our exposure to them.

The fourth nutriment is *consciousness*. Consciousness is not just within us, but also all around us. We consume our own thoughts, and we also consume the thoughts of those around us. It's a bit like secondhand smoke. Consider the family, friends, neighbors, and coworkers with whom you spend your time. Are you picking up some of their suffering and unhelpful mental stories? Are you leaking your mental flotsam onto them?

Mindfulness gives us choice. Without it, our habits will dictate what we consume as the four nutriments—what we eat, what we expose ourselves to, what we deeply desire, and what we think. What we consume not only impacts our own peace of mind, it also creates who we are and influences our words and actions in the world, which live on beyond our lifetime. It's important to consider the effect of all the nutriments we are taking in.

When you practice mindfulness, you can choose to return your attention to the joyful aspects of life. You can find joy in this moment, regardless of the challenges you face. You can find joy in a friend's a joke, a bite of dark chocolate, presenting a meal, or simply a moment of sunshine on a cloudy day.

Easy Peasy *(vegan)*

This vegetable stew is delicious and colorful, a treat for all of the senses. It's also very easy and quick to make.

INGREDIENTS:

  2 cups cooked chickpeas

  1 to 2 tablespoons olive oil

  1 medium onion, diced

  1 large or 2 small garlic cloves, minced

  1 medium carrot, diced

  1 large fresh tomato or canned equivalent, chopped

  1 cup frozen peas

  1 teaspoon garam masala

  ½ teaspoon turmeric

  ½ teaspoon cumin

  salt, pepper, and cayenne, to taste

METHOD:

Heat the olive oil in a skillet over medium heat.

Add onion and cook until transparent.

Add garlic and cook for 1 to 2 minutes.

Add carrots. Cook until they start to soften, stirring regularly.

Stir in tomatoes with juices. If needed, add ⅛ cup water.

Add all spices, and let simmer for several minutes.

Add frozen peas. Turn heat down to low and barely simmer until flavors are blended (about 5 to 10 minutes) and you are ready to enjoy.

Serves 3 to 4 (unless you eat plantains like me, and then: Serves 1).

Olimpia's Homemade Applesauce *(vegan)*

My friend and yoga teacher Olimpia Lee assisted in the kitchen at one of my mindfulness retreats, and we had bought way too many apples. With those that were left, she whipped up a batch of delicious homemade applesauce. Served cold, it is perfect for dessert on a summer evening. In the winter, heat it up or add it to your oatmeal.

INGREDIENTS:

 4 pounds organic apples, peeled, cored, and cut into eighths (sweeter varieties work best)

 1 cup water

 juice of ½ lemon

 ½ to 1 teaspoon cinnamon

 1 teaspoon nutmeg

 ¼ teaspoon salt

METHOD:

Puree the apples with the water in a blender or food processor. Add more water if necessary.

Add apple puree and the rest of the ingredients to a large pot.

Bring to a boil, reduce heat to low, and cover.

Simmer for 10 minutes, stirring frequently.

Serve warm with love.

Serves 10.

Fried Plantains *(vegan)*

This is the recipe I finally figured out that makes delicious sweet plantains. Be sure to be patient with the ripening process. I like them as a sweet dessert, but some people use them more like potatoes as a savory side dish.

INGREDIENTS:

1 to 2 plantains, fully ripe, dark brown on the outside and soft on the inside

coconut, peanut, canola, or similar oil for cooking

METHOD:

Slice the plantains diagonally.

Heat the oil in a saucepan over medium heat.

Once the oil is hot, add the plantains. Let them brown on one side, flip them and brown on the other side, about 3 to 5 minutes each side.

Eat plain, or sprinkle cinnamon and drizzle with honey or maple syrup.

Serves 2.

Kitchen Gathas (Reminders)

Having little reminders around your kitchen or other places where you cook and eat can help you remember your intention to be mindful. In some Buddhist traditions, students memorize many of these reminders in verse, also known as gathas, and use them to keep their minds on the present moment. These gathas come from the Zen tradition of Plum Village. Feel free to use them, modify them, or create your own.

> Breathe, my dear.
> Breathe, it will be all right.

While turning on the faucet:

> Water comes from high mountain sources. Water runs deep in
> the Earth. Miraculously, water comes to us and sustains all life.
> My gratitude is filled to the brim.

While washing your hands before cooking:

> Water flows over these hands.
> May I use them skillfully to preserve our precious planet.

While looking at your empty plate or bowl:

> Looking at this plate (bowl),
> I see how fortunate I am
> to have enough to eat to continue the practice.

> In this food, I see clearly
> the entire universe supporting my existence.

Before eating:

Beings all over the Earth are struggling to live.
I aspire to practice deeply so all may have enough to eat.

With the first taste, I offer joy.
With the second, I help relieve the suffering of others.
With the third, I see others' joy as my own.
With the fourth, I learn the way of letting go.

After eating:

The meal is finished,
and I am satisfied.

While drinking tea:

This cup of tea in my two hands,
mindfulness held perfectly.
My mind and body dwell
in the very here and now.

While washing vegetables:

In these vegetables I see a green sun.
All dharmas (teachings) join together to make life possible.

While taking out the garbage:

In the garbage, I see a rose.
In the rose, I see compost.
Everything is in transformation.
Impermanence is life.

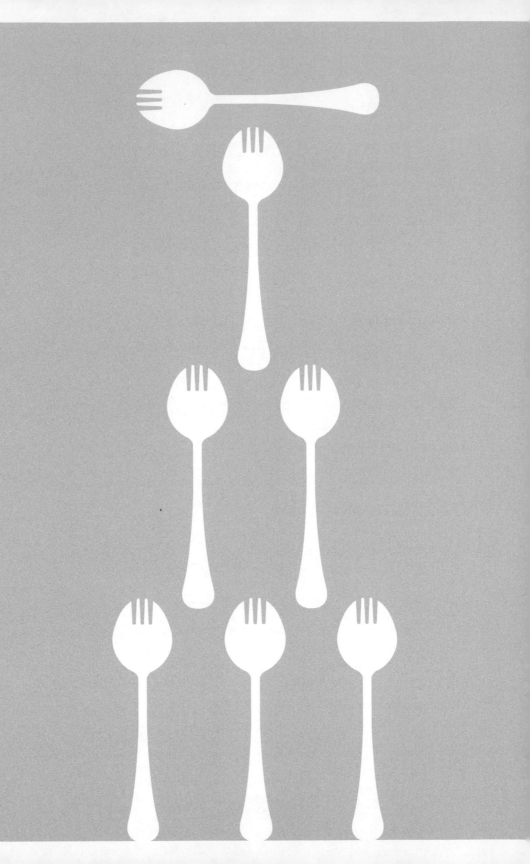

7.

BUILDING FLAVOR

*I am just here, with my eyes, and there is this other being.
If they happen to look into my eyes, they will see that I am
just a shaky being. I have to tolerate that. They may not look.
But if they do, they will see that. They will see the slightly
shy, slightly withdrawing, insecure existence that I am. I
have learnt that that is OK. I do not need to be emotionally
secure and firmly present. I just need to be present. There
are no qualifications for the kind of person I must be.*

—EUGENE GENDLIN, AUTHOR OF *FOCUSING*

Paul and I have just had one of our angry, blaming fights, the kind that start from something as simple as, "Could you please help with the dishes tonight?" and escalates into "What is wrong with you?!" We executed our drama flawlessly: He keeps walking away, and I keep chasing him to try to explain myself. The more I move forward, the more he retreats. He finally walks out of the house to get away from my hounding.

A light bulb seems to go off in my head. I think, "Ohhhhh! I get it now. My husband just doesn't like me as a person." I don't think, "He's angry at me and doesn't like me right now." No, the only thought in my head is, "He doesn't like who I am and he never has." How have I missed this for twenty years?

My mind is saying that he dislikes me in the way you dislike an annoying coworker or the neighbor who always makes awkward and uncomfortable jokes—the kind of dislike that makes you not care enough to even say anything. I am thinking that my husband doesn't want anything to do with me. It's a pretty specific and detailed thought, and in the moment I believe it entirely.

The thought is so powerful and I believe it so thoroughly that I can't think of a single rebuttal to this, in retrospect, irrational mental construction. I get angry about it, I rant, I cry, I eat a peanut butter and jelly sandwich, then another one, I pace around the house and finally collapse on the chair. Nothing helps. My mind is shooting second arrows at the speed of light, creating an ever-larger web of pain. Pretty soon I am convinced that our marriage is a sham because he probably never liked me in the first place. And what will I tell our kids?

LUCKILY, MY MINDFULNESS KICKED IN and I remembered the question Thich Nhat Hanh often poses: "Are you sure?" I was ninety-eight percent sure, but I let the two percent be there. I notice that it was there, and I didn't chase it any further away. And then I wondered, "Who could I ask to help me expand the two percent?" I thought of Dr. Sam, our family therapist. Dr. Sam might be able to shed an objective light on this situation since he seemed to understand our relationship. So I called him. He didn't answer so I left a message asking him if he thought my husband loved me, and if so, could he prove it to me in some way. I would guess that he hadn't gotten *this* message before.

Dr. Sam returned my call right away. First he asked me to explain what had happened, and then he reminded me of some basic facts about our marriage—including the many, many things that Paul had chosen to do because he liked, or maybe even loved, me. Dr. Sam rattled off a very long and varied list of the ways Paul demonstrated his love for me, including staying married for over twenty years and going weekly to couples counseling even though it was emotionally very challenging for him.

After hearing Dr. Sam's long list, my mind began to loosen up. I came up with a few more items myself (like how every night Paul brings home a manila folder of news items he thinks I would be interested in), and I could see that maybe I was being a tiny bit irrational. Clearly it wasn't true that he didn't like me, but something in me, reacting to his walking out the door, had sincerely and fully believed it. My mindfulness practice helped me open up to the possibility that my thought wasn't real, and reaching out to Dr. Sam helped me see past it.

Although I have had many fights and feuds with my husband over the years, this one in particular stands out because it was a moment when I could clearly see one of my sore toes and how my fear of it had been shaping my life.

My Second Arrow

In general, I assume that people don't like me. This idea seems to be part of my hardware—I haven't yet been able to change it the way you can add or delete software apps. I can't remember a time when I didn't think this, though I wasn't aware of the belief for years. When I was young, I thought my parents and siblings didn't like me, and all the way through college, I thought my friends didn't really like me. This unpleasant thought made it less likely that I would experience closeness because I kept telling myself that other people didn't want to be close to me. This second arrow created much of the suffering in my life. For the first three decades of my life, I was confined in a secret isolation created by my complete faith in a faulty thought that I wasn't fully conscious of and that kept me on the hunt for ways to escape the suffering it caused.

Eating disorders such as bulimia, anorexia, and binge eating function like any addiction. In the Anorexics and Bulimics Anonymous "Blue Book" they say, "We came to believe that our eating disorders are addictions, parallel in every respect to alcoholism and drug addiction." It stands to reason, then, that practices that transform drug and alcohol addiction can also help those of us who have difficulty managing our eating behaviors.

Addiction treatment, at least in the US, hasn't been very successful. Dr. Reed Larson's 1985 study on bulimia concluded that the less isolated we are, the less we turn to our emotional eating behaviors.[16] Another researcher, Dr. Bruce Alexander, recognized that rats used in drug addiction research were living isolated lives in tiny cages, and he wondered if perhaps their very isolation impacted whether they succumbed to cocaine addiction.[17] His "Rat Park" experiment demonstrated that rats living alone in cages were easily led into cocaine addiction, while those who were living a relatively happy life in Rat Park (an enclosure two hundred times the size of the cages with plenty of food, wheels and balls for playing, and opportunities for mating) never became regular users. He concluded his research by saying, "Chronic isolation causes people to look for relief. They find temporary relief in addiction to drugs or any of a thousand other habits and pursuits, because addiction allows them to escape from their feelings, to deaden their senses, and to experience an addictive lifestyle as a substitute for a full life."

I am rarely physically distant from family and friends, but because of my implicit belief that none of them really liked me, I have always felt very far away. The more isolated I felt, the more I reached out to deaden my feelings of isolation by eating. When the shame of my binge eating set in, I purged it. Keeping my binge eating secret created another level of distance from the people around me.

When I first started practicing mindfulness, I liked attending retreats, and I found the people around me to be compassionate and friendly. But when I returned home, I still didn't trust other people much, and I avoided finding a meditation community. After practicing meditation for a year on my own without establishing a regular habit, I decided to take the advice I had gotten while on retreat and I tried a meditation group.

I found a local Sangha (community of meditators) that met only two miles from my house in a Sri Lankan Buddhist temple, and I arrived there one Sunday night to meditate. I stepped inside the vestibule. Dozens of pairs of shoes lined the entryway, so I took my own shoes off and left them there with the others. The floor was chilly as I went through into the front hall. There was a door to my immediate right, and a young woman was sitting cross-legged in meditation in front of the door, so I couldn't enter. From a small handwritten sign I realized that I had arrived too late, and that sitting meditation had begun, and I now had to stay outside until the walking meditation. I plopped down on the stairs to wait.

Twenty minutes later, the bell rang inside the meditation hall and the door opened. The woman who had been meditating outside the door stood up and indicated that I could enter. When I got inside, there were about ten people standing beside their cushions waiting to begin walking meditation. I found an empty cushion and stood with my palms joined. There was a ten-foot Buddha statue in an alcove surrounded by flowers and fruit at the front of the hall, which seemed a bit too religious to me at the time. When we finished our walking meditation, we sat for another fifteen minutes and then formed a circle for sharing.

One of the regulars read a passage on forgiveness by Thich Nhat Hanh. I looked around at the other people. Everyone was young and casual, bearded and funky. I was a married mom living in a four-bedroom house in the sleepy, residential Chevy Chase neighborhood of DC. I told myself that I wasn't a good fit for this group. After coming to the Sangha only a few times, I decided not to return—they probably didn't like me anyway, so why bother?

In the Attic

At the end of this first year of faltering mindfulness practice, we went on another mindfulness retreat, and when we got back to DC, I decided to try to visit another meditation community. This time I went to a group that sat every Thursday night in the attic in an old house turned healing center, in a nearby Maryland suburb. I managed to arrive on time, walked up the first two flights of creaky old stairs, went through the attic door, and climbed up an even steeper flight into the meditation hall. There was no Buddha statue—just a cozy group of adults of all ages and appearances sitting in a circle.

As was my habit at the time, I judged everyone based on his or her looks and what they shared in our discussion, which took place after meditation, and I naturally assumed that they didn't like me either. But every Thursday I made the choice to climb those attic stairs and sit down in a circle because I could see how I was being transformed. My meditation became more regular, and I started to have moments of striking clarity when I didn't react out of habit.

One day the senior teacher, Mitchell, asked me to facilitate a discussion. I was so nervous I could barely speak, but I did it. And then he asked me again. I assumed he didn't have time to prepare every week, so he asked some of us to help him—I couldn't imagine he might like me or think I had anything to offer. But I joined the small group that went for tea some nights after our meeting, and I started to feel like I belonged to this group. One night, while walking to our cars, Mitchell told me that he had noticed how much my sharing had changed since I had first joined the Sangha some two years earlier. I was surprised to hear this—I hadn't expected anyone to notice.

Living under the wound caused by my second arrow—that no one liked me—led me to isolate and focus most of my attention on food and weight. I told myself that if only I were thinner or cuter, or had a flatter stomach, people would like me. It wasn't until I learned, through meditation, to sit still with all my inner chatter that I could meet the person underneath and learn to like her.

It's been fifteen years since I started going to Sangha. Just the way it took Dr. Sam to wake me up to the truth that my husband does indeed love me, it took both my meditation and my meditation community to transform my unhealthy relationship to food. Without the ongoing support of a community of like-minded meditators, I would not be writing this book. I'd probably still be caught in a cycle of bingeing and restricting.

The day after Lucile first returned from Ireland, in the grip of her eating disorder, I went to Sangha. When the floor was open for sharing, I thought I would say something about how difficult it had been to see her suffering. I joined my palms together at my heart to indicate that I had something to say, and the other two dozen or so people bowed to me to offer me the floor.

I began to speak, "When my daughter got off the plane yesterday..." but I couldn't hold it together. Seeing the compassionate faces of my mindfulness friends listening attentively broke through my wall of feeling unlovable, and I collapsed into sobs. As I cried, the man next to me, whom I barely knew, reached out to hold my hand, and the entire room sat and witnessed my despair. When I finally caught my breath and was able to continue, I felt as if my pain had been significantly diminished by the mindful listening of the group.

Before that evening I had maintained an emotional distance from the Sangha. I shared what was happening with me, but I also wanted to look good and have it all together. At that moment I didn't have it together. My family was a mess and I didn't know how to solve it. Letting myself look chaotic and emotional in front of the Sangha was a huge step forward in recovering from my self-imposed isolation.

A few years later, I helped start another sitting group on Wednesday mornings at the ridiculous hour of 6:30 a.m. at our new yoga studio. In the winter we arrive and leave in darkness. For some weeks we arrive in darkness and leave at dawn, and on warm summer days I walk to Sangha in the early sunlight.

The members of the Wednesday morning Sangha encouraged me to stay strong and not let Veronica quit her eating disorder treatment program. I had taken Veronica, suffering from depression and binge eating disorder, to a program in the Southwest after a dreadful semester at college. She was willing to go because she was in such terrible emotional distress, but once she was there, she panicked. By the time I got home from the airport, and before they took away her phone, she had sent me more than forty text messages.

On a Tuesday evening not long after she arrived, she begged us to let her leave, saying that the program wasn't going to work, it wasn't for her, it wasn't the right program, and several other fairly compelling arguments. She had agreed to go for one month, and I wasn't sure whether it would be emotionally destructive to make her stay when she didn't want to. I also wondered, though, whether her hesitation was due to her anxiety about facing the discomfort underneath her addictive behaviors.

The next morning, I raised this dilemma with the Sangha after our meditation finished. The five people who were there all gathered around me. Each one said a variation of the same thing: "It's clear to me that she needs to stay." Their comments were based on what they knew about me, our family, mindfulness, and addictions. They were able to see something that I couldn't see about myself: they saw with "Sangha eyes."

As Thich Nhat Hanh says in *Calming the Fearful Mind: A Zen Response to Terrorism*, "In a community, a Sangha, each person trains to see beyond their individual point of view and look with the eyes of collective wisdom, the Sangha eyes." I trusted the collective wisdom of the Sangha, and I told Paul what I thought we should do. The next time Veronica called we told her that she would have to stay at least the thirty days that she originally agreed to. She was furious and wouldn't take our call for several days.

A week later, she told us she was glad to be there, and she ended up staying an extra month because she knew how much it was helping her. Without the Sangha, I would not have known how to make that difficult, important decision to stay the course.

People Are Difficult

I have never found being in any community to be easy. Everyone has different needs, and we don't always get to have our way. Even under the most controlled circumstances, like a silent sitting and walking meditation group, people get on my nerves. I got raging mad at a man who opened a window in an already (to my mind) chilly room, annoyed with the tai chi master who did a dramatic version of walking meditation so slowly that I was nearly forced to give his shoe a flat tire, and frustrated by the woman who told the same story about her thyroid disease at least ten times. Because all of this is happening in silence, however, I have the space to realize that this problem is mine, not theirs. In this mindful space, I am able to use more skillful means to take care of my emotions and communicate my needs. I may still talk with someone about a problem, but I'm no longer likely to blurt out something hurtful like I may have done in the past.

Sharing my experiences and feelings within the safety of the Sangha helped me realize that what I thought of as my own unique dysfunction was "normal." It turns out that many people think other people don't like them (you may be one of them), and lots of us isolate, have kids with serious difficulties, and have wrestled with eating disorders and other addictions.

You may be thinking that a Twelve Step group or group therapy could have been just as helpful, and maybe you're right. But a meditation group offered me skillful conversations as well as the opportunity to learn to be with other people in silence. In silence we don't get to construct a façade with our stories like we can in other kinds of groups. The longer and more often we sit together in silence, the more comfortable we get with being together without our protective armor. It's the combination of the silence and the connection that makes a meditation group so healing. I can't recommend it highly enough. During the Buddha's time, it was the same.

The Buddha's disciple Ananda asked him whether having good spiritual friends to practice with was really half of the spiritual path.[18] Ananda was surprised to hear the Buddha's response: "No, Ananda, having admirable friends is the whole of the path to liberation." Later texts define admirable or "good" friends as those who exhibit "loveableness, esteemableness, venerableness, the ability to counsel well, patience (in listening), the ability to deliver deep discourses, and not applying oneself to useless ends." In my mind this is not limited to people in a meditation community; it includes anyone who is trying his or her best to be kind and to practice mindful speech and deep listening.

Five Ways We Shoot the Second Arrow

Having good friends on the mindfulness path can help us work with our unconscious habits, what the Buddha called "the Five Hindrances." The five traditional hindrances are desire/lust, anger/fear, numbing-out/sleepiness or laziness, worry/guilt, and doubt/ambivalence. These are the five types of "second arrows" with which we shoot ourselves during times of stress.

We all have the habit of employing one or all of these hindrances. The hindrances aren't personal failings, just habitual ways we make our suffering worse by being unwilling to sit with the tenderness and pain of our strong emotions. Usually each person has one or two favorite go-to hindrances; it's helpful to learn which ones you use most, so you can catch yourself before you get too far into it and end up miserable.

Desire/Lust

Desire is the craving for anything that we don't have. All the times I sought out the flavors of Olga's gyros to satisfy my inner emptiness were examples of my desire (and also a form of numbing out, the third hindrance). Desiring food, a new pair of boots, or a different job isn't by itself a problem. But when we think we can relieve our suffering by eating that cake, buying those ankle boots, or getting that promotion, we usually end up disappointed.

Often the Internet is an outlet for my distracted desiring: I'll peruse shopping websites like Amazon, Zappos, Athleta, or gaze at delicious food photos on blogs like Smitten Kitchen. A few months after our standard poodle Gus died, Paul and Louie left for a two-week trip to France, and I was home alone. Before they even got to the airport, I was on my computer looking through pages and pages of rescue dogs. I started sending emails to poodle rescue groups, even though neither Paul nor I were ready for another dog. The truth is, I was really sad that my boys were gone. And I was craving something, anything, to keep me from feeling it. As soon as I recognized this, I sat down on the floor of my office and just cried. Pretty soon I felt a lot better and was able to laugh at myself and my desiring mind. I didn't bring home any dogs that night.

Anger/Fear

Anger is another way we protect ourselves from the vulnerability of the present moment. During the winter break of my sophomore year, my boyfriend Jack and I had an epic, drunken New Year's Eve fight and stumbled home to my parent's house. No one else was awake, so we continued sniping at and blaming each other. In a brief moment of calm, Jack looked at me and said, "I can't do this. I don't want to see you anymore." Although we had fought tooth and nail many times, and I had left him once, this was the first time he had ever broken up with me. I was hammered and in shock, but I knew it was for real. Jack got up and left, and our eighteen-month relationship was over. By the time his car reached the end of our driveway, I was wailing.

I was furious and sad, and I felt abandoned by the only person at that point I ever thought might have actually liked me. I wanted to punish someone for the pain, and the person I decided to punish was myself. I ran through the house (quietly so as not to wake the rest of my family) looking for some kind of pills that I could take to end my life. Luckily for me, my parents were very healthy—they barely took aspirin—and I found nothing that would cause me anything but a stomachache. I thought about slashing my wrists, and tore through medicine cabinets looking for a razor blade, but the men in my family all used electric shavers. I found one of my mom's rusty old disposable razors and tried to cut myself with it, but all I got was a few scratches. I don't know if I was more focused on punishing myself or numbing out, but eventually I became exhausted, climbed under the covers, and disappeared into sleep. I had been lucky, but my anger could have had irreversible consequences that night. When we believe our anger is the truth, we are taken over by its energy and pulled out of the moment. Using our mindfulness practice, we can develop the ability to tolerate our anger without acting out of it.

Numbing-out/Laziness

I am an expert at numbing out. I can numb out with drugs, alcohol, food, overwork, or travel, and I'm sure I could come up with several other techniques if I needed them.

When I was still in graduate school, I lived alone in a tiny apartment on the first floor of a house. One night while I was out very late doing my computer homework, a man broke into my back window and rummaged through all my things. The burglar climbed back out the window when my friend Joe spotted him inside and kicked on my door. Nothing was taken, but when I got home at 2:00 a.m., I was shaken, all alone, and afraid that he might come back. Right then I was struck by a desire for pancakes, and lots of them. When Joe came back to see how I was doing, I said, "Oh, I'm fine now because I just ate a dozen pancakes!"

I was scared and lonely but rather than feel it, I sought out the sweet doughy comfort of pancakes. That night and the next day I felt sick and ashamed. The loneliness and fear didn't go away—I just added a shot of shame to the cocktail.

Worry/Guilt

In 2007 Paul and I dropped our petite seventeen-year-old daughter Lucile off at college before she and I had completely resolved our mother-daughter issues. Her high school years included a lot of yelling and swearing (in both directions), and while we had called a truce, we hadn't yet restitched the fabric where it had torn. My husband drove her to school in Florida, and I flew down with just Jamie, because both Veronica and Louie were at a weight-loss camp.

After moving all her belongings into her dorm room and attending a short parent orientation, we were invited to a barbecue on the patio between the college café and the administration buildings. Lucile, though quiet, seemed happy to be there, and we tried to keep a comfortable conversation going over ribs and salad. I worried about what Lucile's life would be like at college without us and with a roommate who kept a rat and a smelly ferret under her bed. My worry and guilt were the second arrows that kept me from feeling my grief and from being present for what Lucile was really feeling.

We met another family dropping off their child, and had just finished eating when Lucile abruptly announced, "It's time for you to go." No other parents were leaving, but apparently she was ready. We walked her back to her dorm room, where we said good-bye to her and returned to our rental car. Paul was happy to get an early start to the airport, but I was grieving the sudden detachment from my firstborn. Caught in my worries, I missed the opportunity for a heartfelt good-bye with Lucile.

Lucile came home for a mid-semester break in October, and it wasn't until I dropped her back at the airport to return to college that I felt the full weight of my sadness. I cried all the way home, grieving the loss of time with a child with whom I was just starting to heal old wounds. Once I became familiar with my grief, I was much more present to Lucile and to the rest of my family. Like the other hindrances, worry and guilt trap us in the past and the future with no connection to the reality of what we are feeling and needing in the present moment. Had I been in touch with my grief, rather than worrying and feeling guilty, I wouldn't have missed the chance for a more intimate connection with Lucile.

Doubt/Ambivalence

In calling doubt a hindrance, the Buddha is referring especially to our doubts about ourselves and our spiritual practice. Am I really getting anywhere? Is this practice really helping me to transform? Should I be meditating in a different way? I have spent considerable time searching for various ways to practice (different religions, different styles of meditation, different meditation groups) rather than sinking into one practice deeply. During a retreat, the meditation teacher Phillip Moffitt once told us that our practice would be more beneficial if we chose one path and followed it. He said that if we never choose a path, we will never get anywhere. If we choose a path and it's not right, we can always try another one, but if we never commit to a path, we never even get started. This makes sense to me.

Doubting takes us into our minds and away from our senses. We start obsessing about whether we should or shouldn't have eaten or said something, wondering whether we are transforming fast enough, or if we are eating healthy today, whether we will return to our unhealthy eating tomorrow. All this doubting prevents us from living in the present moment ,and doesn't help us solve any of our problems, either.

Keep Shooting

I could tell a story about myself using all the hindrances at once. Paul is late for dinner, again. I've been trying to work all day, and managing the kids before coming home to put dinner on the table. He is expected at 6:30, but calls at 6:35 to say he is just leaving. I have to hold down the family, already milling about the dinner table, for another twenty-five minutes. First there is anger: I want to blame Paul for everything—it's his fault that we have four kids all basically the same age, that I have too much to do because he doesn't help enough, and that he is late. Argh!

Then, there is the worry and guilt: I shouldn't blame him, I'm not very nice, and I get mad too easily. He's trying really hard, blah blah blah. Then the doubt hits: Maybe I just married the wrong person. There's someone out there who would come home on time every night. Or maybe we shouldn't have had so many kids, or maybe we shouldn't try to eat dinner together. Maybe I should meditate more or find a different practice. Maybe…

Then self-doubt shows up. If only I had planned this better. I should have guessed that he would be late again. If only I had planned for a later dinner, or made something that wouldn't get cold. Did I forget to tell him dinner was at 6:30?

He's still not home at 6:50, so desire sets in. I'll feel better with a bite of pasta. Well, actually a small bowl of pasta will tide me over. And a piece of garlic toast, or the whole loaf. I'd better have some chocolate to top it off. Then there is numbing out: I don't want to think about how much I just ate or how upset I am, so I'll just lie down and rest until he gets here. But then guilt returns: Why did I eat so much? Now I'll be fat and no one will like me. Well, they already don't like me, so what difference does it make? And on and on it goes.

The Five Hindrances are simply the five categories of ways we shoot ourselves with the second arrow to avoid taking care of our tender, raw hearts. Underneath all our bingeing, fighting, sleeping, guilt-tripping, and self-doubting we are hurting. Some part of us is in pain, but we don't want to feel it. Of course we don't, because it hurts!

Growing Up

The practice of mindfulness instructs us to welcome our shadows and vulnerabilities. The more we practice sitting still with what arises, the more stability we have to hold difficult emotions. It's like we are training ourselves to grow up enough to hold our wounded child. Ann Weiser Cornell, author of *The Radical Acceptance of Everything: Living a Focusing Life*, and Barbara McGavin, her Inner Relationship Focusing (IRF) cocreator, call this our "Self-in-Presence." It's who we are when we are really and completely present for what is.

Cornell describes Self-in-Presence as "the alternative to being in a reactive state. Self-in-Presence is a state of calm, curious, accepting, warm attention. Turning with this kind of attention toward an emotional state results in significant relief in itself, and at the same time opens up a state in which a felt sense can form, creating new possibilities of thought, feeling, and behavior."

Learning how to care for our wounded parts with gentleness also teaches us how to both give and receive that kind of care with others. The more we befriend ourselves, the more we can befriend others. The more we connect with others, the more we can connect with ourselves. They are two sides of the same coin.

During the time I was learning to be with emotions that I had avoided for decades, I went on several ten-day silent mindfulness retreats. At those retreats we didn't speak at all, except for two fifteen-minute conversations each week with a teacher. We didn't have eye contact with anyone or use phones or email. Each day we alternated between sitting meditation and walking meditation from 6:00 a.m. until 9:30 p.m. with just three short meal breaks, one afternoon rest, and a one-hour Dharma talk in the evening.

As I focused on my in-breath and out-breath for days at a time, I opened a space for all my unheard and unseen emotions to finally be known. Memories and feelings bubbled up during every meditation period. Some of the feelings were light enough to float by, but some brought waves of mourning or regret. At the end of each retreat, I felt that I had given those wounded parts of myself just what they needed, and I had more energy and attention available for the other people in my life. The more love I gave myself, the more love I had to give to others.

Growing up on the inside is like growing up as a child—we have to trip and fall before we can walk. It wasn't easy for me to change my patterns of isolation. My friend and meditation teacher Mitchell, from my first real Sangha, helped me get there. We have very different styles, and we drive each other a little crazy, but ours has been one of the relationships that has helped me grow up the most. In her book *Worst Enemy, Best Teacher*, my friend Deidre Combs says, "We may not like them and we may justly fear them, but we absolutely need our opponents... Our adversaries show us who we are by holding up a contrasting side."

At lunch one day, Mitchell told me that I didn't play well with others unless I could be in charge. This was partly true, but I was offended (and hurt) and attacked him in response. I vented to a friend about my frustration with Mitchell. She told me I should just let the relationship go if it was that onerous. I was starting to understand that some of the judgments I had about other people were coming from my own insecurities, and I wanted to experiment with this relationship. If I stuck with it, would I see that some of my judgments were wrong, and would I develop the ability to transform other difficult relationships? We weren't best friends, so there was less at stake. Also, Mitchell was a skilled mindfulness practitioner and was willing to tolerate his own hurts and frustrations without ditching our friendship.

Living on Ice Mountain

During this same period of time, I became an aspirant to ordain in the Order of Interbeing, a community of monastics and laypeople established by Thich Nhat Hanh. Ordination meant that in addition to practicing with The Five Mindfulness Trainings, I would also be aspiring to practice The Fourteen Mindfulness Trainings. The Fourteen Mindfulness Trainings aren't distinct from The Five Mindfulness Trainings; they just describe the path in more depth. To do this, I made a commitment to a specific practice community (Plum Village)—kind of like a marriage.

To receive The Fourteen Mindfulness Trainings, I had to work with a mentor. I was assigned to Mitchell. We took long walks around the city together discussing and debating the trainings, and the challenges and joys we each were experiencing in our families, our work, and our mindfulness practices.

We knocked heads nearly every time we had a conversation. We tried so many ways to work with our conflicts. For a while Mitchell and I only emailed because it gave me time to pause between hearing him and responding. We started each conversation with the full intent to practice deep listening and nonviolent communication, and though it often devolved into gentle bickering, I deepened my ability to listen, especially to things I didn't want to hear. Most important, we agreed that although this was hard work, we respected and cared about each other enough to stay friends.

One day on retreat in Plum Village, Mitchell was getting on a bus to begin walking the Camino de Santiago in Spain—I wouldn't see him for three months. I suddenly realized how he had helped me learn that I could feel cared for and connected to someone even while a big part of me wanted to bolt. Although I still don't agree with him all of the time, we are both committed to deepening our understanding of mindfulness and helping people learn to practice. His commitment to our friendship was a gift that helped me transform my habit of isolating myself. I ran over to where he was boarding the bus, gave him a big hug, and told him how much he meant to me.

Mitchell and I continue to disagree and we continue to stay friends. Through our commitment to our mindful friendship, we have created a relationship based on deep mutual respect and the willingness to always trust that the other person is doing their best—rather than a friendship based on shared experiences, similar tastes, or agreement on everything. This is what we all need: Sangha—other people whom we can trust to sit with us in silence and grow with us. Without a community, we are just meditating on top of a mountain of ice—isolated and alone. Thich Nhat Hanh often reminds us that the test of our practice isn't how we sit on the cushion, it's how we are in relationship to others.

Belly Rolls

One of the wonderful side effects of practicing mindful eating and cooking is a healthier body and weight. I don't weigh myself anymore, but I wear nearly the same size I did when I started meditating on a regular basis and sitting with a Sangha. Granted, my shape has changed as I've aged, and I've gone up and down ten pounds a few times. But to be honest, I have stopped caring much about my weight. I continue to exercise nearly every day because I enjoy it and it makes me feel more energetic.

I can actually look straight at my belly rolls (that now divide both horizontally and vertically because of my C-section scar) when I'm naked and think, "Hello there, belly." I'm not excited about how it looks, but at least I'm not verbally abusing it anymore. Sometimes I wish I had the actress Jennifer Aniston's body, but more often I think, "This is the body I've got and it's working pretty well." I have even taken my belly out of hiding a few times on topless beaches (far away from anyone who knows me).

The first arrow is the truth that my body is aging. I don't need to add a second arrow of suffering. The body I have is five feet five inches tall with hips and legs like a preteen boy, a belly like the laughing Buddha, boobs like Dolly Parton (at the age she is now), and as I was told by a massage therapist once, I have a neck like an NFL player. I have never, even when I was just slightly more than one hundred pounds, had a completely flat belly unless I was lying flat on my back. And yet this body has done pretty much everything I have ever asked it to do.

Girls and women continue to face more fat-shaming than boys and men. In an article in *Esquire*, Chris Jones described the actor Vince Vaughn's belly pouring out from his unbuttoned shirt as "great golden acreage" and he is referred to with affection as "the biggest man in the room."[19] In contrast, actress Melissa McCarthy was described by the highly regarded film critic, Rex Reed, as "tractor-sized," and "female hippo."[20] We all lose out if our young (and old) women waste valuable time and energy trying to reach an unattainable goal or succumb to shame about their weight.

I hope that our culture will find a way to stop overfocusing on body shape, especially women's. I wince at the pressure facing my girls to maintain a certain body shape. I remember how demoralizing it was for me when I was trying to beat my hunger and my body into submission. I never thought I looked the way I should.

The goal of mindful cooking and eating is so much more than physical well-being. As my relationship with food has become more peaceful, food can now be a healing force rather than something forbidden, avoided, or despised. Dissatisfaction with myself, my body, and my life will continue to arise, but I now have the ability to see it for what it is, and not let it take over my life. Impermanence reminds me that whatever difficulties arise will also pass, and whatever happiness I have now, I should savor to the fullest. Through the truth of interdependence, I know that the food I prepare and eat is not separate from me and I am not separate from other people.

The ultimate goal is finding contentment in whatever is happening right now. To reach that goal you need a clear intention to practice and an awareness of obstacles that may be in your way. Finding a safe mindfulness community will help shine the light on your sore toes, boost your practice, and make the journey more fun.

When you do get tripped up by any hindrance, as we all will, gently remind yourself of your intentions, and keep going. There is no moment at which you will suddenly be done with this practice; but like playing the violin, you start out scratchy but sound better each day.

Your intentions arise from your own inner wisdom, not from outside of yourself. Though you wouldn't guess it by listening to product advertisements, there is really nothing, other than food, that you need to buy, own, think, or learn to begin your journey of mindful cooking and eating. You don't need fancy kitchen equipment or even a meditation cushion to get started.

Step into your kitchen, or sit down with your food. Notice what you see, hear, taste, smell, think, or feel. Take a mindful breath. Notice what comes up in your body-mind. If you find yourself hooked by self-doubt ("I can't do this") or numbing out ("Let me just eat already"), turn toward this feeling rather than away. Underneath the second arrow of each hindrance is a wound from the first arrow. What hurts? What needs your love?

As soon as you turn toward your tender heart, you become your grown-up self, caring for your wounded child. In its presence you know what you want to eat, how to enjoy cooking and eating, and how to eat without guilt and shame. When I eat from my grown-up self, I feel like the woman in the movie *Chocolat* when, describing chocolate seashells, she says, "And it *melts*, God forgive me, it melts ever so slowly on your tongue, and tortures you with pleasure."

You can start any time.

Camille's Mushroom Barley Soup (vegan)

Camille, who's been my friend for more than twenty years, loves to cook for other people. Maybe it's her Italian heritage, or maybe it's because she comes from a family of eleven kids. She says that preparing food for her family and friends is more meaningful than any material gifts she could give them. Cooking for others reminds her of the fact that she has the means to cook healthy food, so it makes her feel grateful. And she makes food that she enjoys and wants to share with her loved ones. She says, "In a way it goes from my heart and stomach to theirs." She makes me a pot of this soup whenever I'm sick in bed or I just need some love.

INGREDIENTS:

1 cup uncooked pearled barley

8 to 9 cups vegetable broth, canned, boxed, or homemade

olive oil

2 onions, chopped

1 or 2 garlic cloves, chopped

8 to 16 ounces fresh mushrooms, sliced

one large bag (or bag and a half) of fresh loose spinach

salt and pepper, to taste

1 bay leaf

fresh thyme (optional)

METHOD:

Sauté the onions and chopped garlic in olive oil on medium-low heat until about halfway cooked or transparent.

Add the cleaned and sliced mushrooms.

Add a pinch of salt and a pinch of pepper.

Cook until mushrooms and onions are thoroughly cooked, even crisp.

In a large soup pot, add broth, mushrooms/onions, garlic, bay leaf, spinach, salt and pepper, barley, and thyme (if including), and bring to a boil on medium heat.

Turn heat down to simmer and cook with the top on until barley is tender (anywhere from 60 to 90 minutes).

If it's too thick, add more broth—if not thick enough, add some precooked barley.

Serves 8 to 10.

Warming Sweet Potato Chickpeas à la Jon & Jim
(vegan)

My nephews Jon and Jim are both vegetarians who love to cook and share vegetarian recipes. Jon was with us at Plum Village during the heat-wave summer. This dish was taught to me by Jim, who learned it from Jon. It's destined to be a family recipe for generations, and it's delicious.

INGREDIENTS:

1 medium sweet potato peeled and diced into bite-sized cubes

1 can chickpeas (15 ounces)

1 teaspoon cumin seeds

1 teaspoon ground coriander

2 tablespoons olive oil or coconut oil

1 small bunch spinach (optional)

salt to taste

cayenne pepper to taste

optional: sauté 1 small onion, very thinly sliced, and add it to the sweet potato cubes

METHOD:

Gently and slowly roast cumin seeds, coriander, and salt in medium
  nonstick skillet at medium-high heat until they begin to give off a
  nice aroma.

Add olive oil and sweet potato cubes and mix well, until sweet potatoes are
  coated with the cumin mixture.

Cover completely and reduce heat to low-medium.

Stir the sweet potatoes often and cook them until they're soft (about
  30 minutes).

Drain and add chickpeas. Mix well.

If adding spinach, wash it and add to the pan. Stir and cover until spinach
  is just wilted.

Serve with the grain of your choice, and sprinkle cayenne as desired
  for heat.

Serves 2 to 3.

Sangha Potluck Tofu (*vegan*)

This is the perfect simple dish to make when going to a vegetarian pot-luck with your admirable friends. It's full of protein, which is something that most veggie potlucks are in need of, but it's also just really good and satisfying. Get crazy with the marinade. My Sangha friend David always uses Soy Vay.

INGREDIENTS:

> 14 ounces extra firm tofu
>
> ½ to 1 teaspoon olive, sesame, or other oil

FOR MARINADE:

> Ginger teriyaki sauce, barbecue sauce, soy sauce, or any favorite marinade

METHOD:

Drain and dry the tofu.

Cut the tofu into slices or cubes.

Marinade the tofu for 5 minutes to 1 hour or overnight.

Coat the bottom of a saucepan with oil on medium-high heat.

Place the tofu in the pan and cook it until it's brown, about 5 to 7 minutes.

Flip the tofu and brown other side.

Top with the remaining marinade and serve.

Serves 6.

Mindful Ways to Avoid a Binge

Sometimes we can feel a binge coming on, and we have a moment or two before we reach for the food, and sometimes we become aware of what we're doing in the middle of compulsive eating. This isn't about simply avoiding eating a lot. It's about learning how to take care of the parts in you that are warring over food, so that you can end the battle.

These ideas come from my practice of Inner Relationship Focusing (IRF), which I think of as a way to develop the ability to be with and care for our strong emotions. Along with my mindfulness meditation, IRF has been a very important part of my journey toward peace with food, because it has helped me learn to be with all my compulsive parts. Find out more at www.focusingresources.com.

If you have a moment of clarity when the part of you that doesn't want to eat is asking for help, here are a few suggestions that have worked for me:

1. *The* most important thing: Don't get angry at yourself. Even if getting angry at yourself is a natural impulse, in the long run it will induce more compulsive behavior than it stops.

2. Say hello to the small voice in you that doesn't want to binge. Expand on it. Describe it to yourself. For example, say, "I can feel that something in me doesn't want to do to do this. It knows that I will feel sick later." Or, "There's part of me that doesn't want to feel ashamed later, but it feels hopeless because it thinks that I am going to binge anyway." See if you can get to the feeling of this part of you in your body. And see if you can get even a small sense of why it doesn't want to eat. You aren't deciding not to eat, you are just taking a moment to hear the other side.

3. Tell the part of you that wants to eat that you can eat, but you'd like to have a short conversation first. If possible, leave the food area and sit down somewhere quiet (the bathroom has always been a great quiet spot for me). Listen to the part that really wants to eat. Find out where it lives in your body and why it wants to eat. Gently see if you can get to the underlying feeling it is having (e.g., sadness, fear, anger). Empathize with it. "Of course you're mad, that jerk made you work late again!" You are the compassionate parent taking care of the upset child. Keep listening and

empathizing as long as you can. Be sure not to send the message that you are listening to try to get rid of it—you aren't. You are just listening to that part of yourself because you care.

4. If you are able to do so, write about it. Write down what you want to eat, and the reasons why. Write about the part of you that doesn't want to eat too.

5. See if you can hold both parts of you—the one that doesn't want to eat and the one that does—like two little babies (twins!) or two delicate birds. You can imagine that you have one in each hand and that you are the loving mother who will take care of both of them.

6. You can practice this even in the midst of a compulsive eating episode. The one who wants to eat is getting his or her way, but you can still be there compassionately caring for the part that didn't want to eat. And vice versa. If you don't eat, take special care of the part that really wanted to. That part may be feeling helpless.

7. Check back in with these parts and let them know that you are here for them, even when a binge is not at hand. Consider checking in with them each day.

8. Continue to draw or write about this. I like to draw pictures of the parts of myself because I learn something about them when I see how they look and how they relate to each other.

Hugging Meditation

You likely already know how to give and receive a hug. Sometimes hugs, like food, are over before we even know what happened. Hugging meditation is extended hugging, so we have time to take in the hug and the person we are hugging. It's nice to practice this with our family and close friends, to really savor our relationship and to remember these sweet but impermanent moments. It's really simple.

1. Have direct eye contact with the person you are about to hug. Both of you are committed to making this mindful hug happen.

2. Step in toward each other and embrace gently but firmly. Think Grandma hug. Don't compress their diaphragm, but don't treat them as though they have a brittle bone disease (unless they do!). Think about the Middle Way when choosing your squeeze depth.

3. Now that you're in there, breathe. Nice and slowly. If possible, sync your breathing up with the other person's, but don't struggle too hard to make it happen. This is a relaxing practice. During your first in-breath and out-breath, sense your own body. Feel your feet on the ground and your body touching theirs, and just notice how great it is to be alive and in relationship.

4. On your second breath, notice the other person. Feel them in your arms, notice how they smell, and bring to mind all the nice things about this person.

5. On your third breath, become aware of how lucky you are to have this particular person in your life. It's a rare pleasure to engage with someone who loves us enough to want to be this close to us for three luxurious breaths. Consider how your lives have been interwoven over the past years or even just days. Celebrate your relationship. If you have time left over, consider what this relationship will be in two hundred years—it's a good reminder of the impermanence of everything.

6. After about the third breath it's time to let go. We can't hold on forever. Sometimes a little extra squeeze before letting go is nice. Like you're saying, "This is just good-bye for now."

Important note: Please don't surprise anyone with hugging meditation. My husband tells the story about the time (before he knew about hugging meditation) when he was greeting someone from our mindfulness community, and they held on to him there for three breaths while he was thinking, "What the hell is going on?!"

8.

BREAKING BREAD

Everyone should be born into this world happy and loving everything. But in truth it rarely works that way. For myself, I have spent my life clamoring toward it. Halleluiah, anyway I'm not where I started.

—MARY OLIVER, "HALLELUIAH"

I'm in my early twenties, watching my eighty-four-year-old maternal grandmother, Lucile, bake bread. We're in her kitchen. As soon as you step into Grandma's house, you are in her kitchen, a twenty-foot by twenty-foot room with a door on each of the four walls. Her stove is along the far wall. We are working on a table just to the left of the stove. I take notes so that I can make the same bread and share it with the other grandkids.

Grandma doesn't use a recipe. Making bread is a humble task that she has been performing for at least five decades. It involves only a few ingredients but lots of hard work. She forgoes any time- or energy-saving tricks like a Cuisinart (which I use) to knead the bread or a breadmaker, which does all the work.

Everything is determined by her senses. Her eyes decide if the yeast is alive enough to rise the dough and if she has the right amount of salt and flour; her hands feel for the proper texture of the dough ball, which lets her know that it is ready to be formed; her nose guides her to the oven when it's time to monitor the final moments of baking; her ears can tell, when she thwacks the bottom of the loaf with her fingertips, whether the bread has baked long enough; and the epic moment when her mouth tastes the first piece of bread and convinces her that her work is done: the bread is soft, warm, chewy, and buttery. Scrumptious.

I am the first person to ask to learn the secret of the Hemenger bread, and Grandma is flustered by my attention. She says, "Goodness gracious, Annie. Do you really want to watch your old Grandma make bread?" She doesn't see why anyone would want to know how to make this simple, utilitarian bread that, for her, is as unexciting as vacuuming the living room or writing thank-you notes.

Even so, she doesn't rush through it like I might. She chuckles when I ask her how much honey she adds to the yeast mixture. As if she would know. There are no specifics to record, so I write down general notes and measurements based on what I see her adding.

Her intuition at this point is always right, since she has been making the same bread for—basically—ever.

I tell her that I expected a more formal demonstration, and we laugh as she plunges her hand into the water to make sure it is the right temperature. With the water, yeast, and honey mixture in her big ceramic bowl, she begins the process of adding flour. This is where it really gets inventive. She tells me, "You add until you can't add any more." "Oh really," I think to myself. "I can always add more." It reminds me of my life, how I am already, at this young age, adding more and more to my schedule. First a full-time job I detest, then a husband (whom I love), then a new house, then a full-out do-it-yourself construction project on that house, and pretty soon I will be pregnant. Grandma seems to have a better sense of when to stop adding than I do.

Each time she dumps flour into the mix from her metal cup, Grandma uses a wooden spoon to stir the now glue-like sticky contents of the bowl. I start to think the dough must be ready, but she continues to add flour and stir. Another cup of flour and the contents are pulling together into a bolus that sticks irregularly to the sides of the bowl. I think it must be ready to knead now. Not yet. Another quarter cup, and the ball of dough is barely sticking to the sides. Grandma announces that it's time.

She dumps the soccer ball-sized sphere of dough onto the part of the table that she had earlier dusted with flour. She says, "Now we have to really work hard," with a false kind of seriousness that makes us both laugh. My grandma is soft and huggable with a honey-sweet voice, but she is no wimp. She took care of her sick husband for a couple of decades, helping him get around in a wheelchair until his prostate cancer spread to his brain, which required that he lie flat on his back in a hospital bed in the middle of their living room. Then she and her community of friends made sure all his needs were met, including daily changing, bathing, and shaving. One of my lasting images of Grandma is how she sat next to his bed for hours reading the newspaper aloud to him.

MENTALLY, GRANDMA WAS FEISTY TOO. She always spoke up when she heard neighbors make racist comments, taught special education in a one-room schoolhouse, and rode in the annual July Fourth Parade once as her town's Citizen of the Year. When I became a vegetarian, she was furious, believing that my mom had convinced me to take on an unhealthy practice.

So Grandma had no trouble beating up a five-pound ball of dough. Even with arthritis in nearly every knuckle, she repeatedly pushed the dough down with the heel of her hand, folded the dough back over itself, and pushed it forward again. She used her whole body weight, rather than her arms alone, to push the dough to keep from injuring oneself. She worked the dough for close to ten minutes, adding flour when the dough seemed to "need it." Then she stopped and said, "It feels right." Since she couldn't tell me exactly what that meant, I felt it myself. It was dense and firm, but not hard, with very little stickiness remaining.

She oiled a second even larger ceramic bowl and set the dough ball carefully in the oil, flipped it over so both sides were oiled, and covered it with a towel. She placed the bowl on her kitchen table, which was near a hot-water radiator that would keep the dough warm while it rose. We were done for now. Then Grandma and I drove to the grocery store in her white Ford Escort, and when we got back, she talked on the phone with my Uncle Bill. Then we sat down in her living room to read.

After about two hours had passed, Grandma checked on our dough. I was surprised to see that it had nearly doubled in size, and was even more surprised when she sucker-punched the dough right in the center. It deflated immediately. "There," she said. And we went back to reading.

Some hours later, we went back into the kitchen. Grandma turned on her ancient oven, setting it to 350 degrees. The dough ball had risen to about the same size it had been before she socked it earlier. She pulled it back out of the bowl onto the floury table before separating it into five relatively equal pieces. She rolled one out like a wide Play-Doh snake (and I finally get its name: "play dough"). After rolling one snake, she tucked its ends under and placed it, tucked sides down, in a pre-buttered and floured bread pan. She did this for all five pieces.

My mother contested this next step, years later after Grandma died. She claimed that her mother always brushed the top of the bread with a well-beaten egg before it went into the oven. Either Grandma forgot to do that on this day, or I forgot to write it down, but I don't remember seeing it happen. Either way, she put all five loaves into the hot oven to cook. She said it would take about thirty minutes, but we never looked at the clock. Instead, when we started smelling the bread from the living room, which may have been half an hour later, we went into the kitchen. Grandma warned me that opening the oven had a deleterious effect on the bread if it wasn't ready, so we waited until we could really smell it before we opened the oven. She quickly grabbed one of the loaves, pulled it onto the counter next to the oven, and shut the door to protect the other loaves.

The rounded top of the loaf was a light golden brown. Grandma tipped it upside down on the counter so that the loaf fell partway out of the pan. She tapped on the bottom of the loaf and it made a slightly hollow sound. "That," she said, "means it's done." I was so excited—until now, I had only had Grandma's homemade bread fresh from the oven on one or two other occasions, when she happened to have baked it on a day that we were visiting. When it was cool enough to slice without crushing it, she cut me a piece and spread butter in chunks onto the bread. Each chunk melted in place, leaving puddles of butter on steaming hot bread. It was delicious.

Baking bread was simple but not easy. It was a ritual, one that required Grandma to be present throughout the process and in touch with all her senses. It was, frankly, a lot like meditation. And, like meditation, it's not done for us alone. Of course, Grandma enjoyed eating her own bread. But most of her bread was eaten by her family and friends. It was an expression of her love. Grandma's bread was all about presence and community.

Four Ennobling (Not Enabling) Truths

All the difficulties we encounter in life are what the Buddha called the First Noble Truth of suffering. They're not personal failings, they're just unavoidable aspects of living in this world. The only choice we have is how we respond to them. Meditation teacher Phillip Moffitt says, "In surrendering to the ups and downs of your life, you discover the truth of your inner dignity."[21]

When I encountered mindfulness practice, I started to understand how I was making my suffering worse with all my negative stories and my constant seeking of pleasure and avoiding pain. This is the Second Noble Truth: There's a reason we are suffering. Whenever I felt pain, I ate too much, became angry or afraid, shut down with alcohol, drugs, or sleep, and worried, felt guilt, or obsessed about it. These were the second arrows of my suffering, and none of them made me hurt less; in fact, they made my suffering worse.

The Third Noble Truth reminds us that change is possible. No matter who we are or what our addictions might be, every one of us is capable of transforming ourselves and generating a peaceful life. Everyone wants to feel at ease and content; none of us wants to suffer. We keep choosing to binge, get drunk, or starve ourselves because we don't know a better way to meet our needs.

As Marshall Rosenberg says, "Behind every action, however ineffective, tragic, violent, or abhorrent to us, is an attempt to meet a need." Mindfulness offers us a path to meeting our needs for a peaceful relationship with food. It may not be an easy path, but it is well worth traveling because we won't only learn to restore our relationship with food, we'll learn how to create peace in every aspect of our lives.

The Fourth Noble Truth is the Buddha's recipe for generating this peace. He called it the Eightfold Path.

Baking Peace

Like my grandma's bread recipe, there are only a few ingredients in the Eightfold Path. And, like baking bread, it's simple but not easy. It's not a recipe you can follow with your eyes closed. Creating a peaceful life requires seeing, tasting, hearing, smelling, and feeling in each moment. And we also need familiarity with our sixth sense—our mind—in order to recognize when we are adding "shoulds," "if onlys," or "the right ways" to our mixture. Adding these second arrows is likely to send our peacefulness up in flames.

Making peace—and baking bread—takes time and effort, and you have to know when enough is enough, when you "can't add any more." If we push too hard we will hurt ourselves, or risk over-kneading the bread. If it becomes a chore, we won't keep doing it. Thich Nhat Hanh's wisdom in his 1991 book *Peace Is Every Step* applies just as well to baking bread: "We sit in meditation to help us cultivate peace, joy, and nonviolence, not to endure physical strain or to injure our bodies."

We also have to know when to bake alone and when to share with others, when to practice on our meditation cushion and when to be with a community of friends. Thich Nhat Hanh goes on to say, "Sometimes, we can use meditation as a way of hiding from ourselves and from life, like a rabbit going back to his hole. Doing this, we may be able to avoid some problems for a while, but when we leave our 'hole,' we will have to confront them again."

Like baking bread, mindfulness works on its own schedule. We might see some results from our mindfulness practice right away—maybe we aren't choosing to binge as often or we enjoy making dinner a little bit more—but other aspects may take more time. If we practice regularly, however, our new mindful relationship with food will eventually become second nature.

The Five Mindfulness Trainings (see Appendices on page 233) are a concrete expression of the Eightfold Path, offered by the Buddha to people who simply wanted to find peace but weren't interested in becoming a monk or reaching some kind of exalted state. Like you, me, and everyone else, they just wanted to be happy.

What I love most about the Eightfold Path is its practicality. Like a recipe, it's a list of suggestions. You can do with it what you want without being told you'll go to hell or be ostracized. The Buddha, like a chef, was a scientist at heart. He experimented with the mind the same way a chef experiments in the kitchen. The Buddha told his students not to do anything blindly just because he said it—he told them to try his suggestions out for themselves. If they suffer less as a result, they should keep doing it. If they suffer more, they shouldn't do it.

My Grandma couldn't specify measures or times because there were so many variables—the health of the yeast, sweetness of the honey, denseness of the flour, strength of your kneading, oven temperature variability, altitude, etc. I can't offer you any measures or times for the Eightfold Path either. There are just as many variables as baking bread: how often you meditate, whether you have supportive friends and community, how extensive your conditioning is, the culture you live in, the teachers you study with, and more. What I do know for sure is that if you stay on the path, you will find peace.

The Eightfold Path

1. Wise Approach
Get to know the Three Contemplations (see chapter 4). Sometimes life sucks, nothing lasts, and we're all in this together. When you really internalize these, they self-generate gratitude and compassion—for yourself and everyone else. Sometimes the bread doesn't rise, when we eat the bread it's gone, and it takes the whole cosmos to create a loaf of bread.

2. Wise Intention
Look into what motivates your life. Are you trying to get somewhere or prove something, or do you want to find true peace? Consider what you want out of your life, and then break that down into bite-sized pieces. How do I

move toward my intention today? Write it down each morning. Think of it throughout the day. Live it. Only by setting intentions for your practice will you transform these teachings into a lamp helping to guide you toward more happiness. With your intentions, your experiences can leave this page and support your ability to be more mindful in your kitchen and your life. Without your intentions, these words will stay on the page, and you won't effect these changes in your life.

3. Wise Mindfulness

Forget the recipe. Feel your way. Breathe in… breathe out. You have arrived; you are home. Live in your senses—see, feel, hear, smell, and taste your life. One of The Fourteen Mindfulness Trainings reminds us, "The knowledge we presently possess is not changeless, absolute truth. Truth is found in life." Can you live completely for just this one breath?

4. Wise Effort

How much kneading does your dough need? When you're inspired, go for it; when you're tired, rest. There's no place to get to. As Alan Watts says in his book *The Wisdom of Insecurity*, life is like a dance and "when you are dancing you are not intent on getting somewhere." But, if you've given up, you're not dancing. Have fun.

5. Wise Speech

Consider what is going out of your mouth as well as what is coming in. Our words live forever in the hearts and minds of those who hear them. What we say can give us valuable clues to our intentions and our mind states; is it possible to speak only when you know it's important information, it's the right time, and it's the truth?

6. Wise Action

It's hard to believe, but everything we do has an impact. If we add too much salt, our bread will be awful. If the yeast is fresh and we knead it long enough, it will rise. We don't have full control over the outcome, but we always have an impact. Our actions and reactions are the only things we can control, but only if we are aware we are acting. If we practice mindfulness, we are more aware of what we are doing and so can act in ways we feel good about.

7. Wise Livelihood

Baking bread is a lovely way to give back. But it's certainly not the only way. Does your work (paid or unpaid) contribute to your own happiness and to the benefit of the world? How does your work make you feel?

8. Wise Concentration/Bliss

You've come this far, so it's time to enjoy the fruits of your practice. After pulling the steaming-hot loaf of bread out of the oven, you cut a slice, slather it with butter or vegan margarine, and stuff it in your mouth. Let the butter slide down your chin, roll your eyes back, and moan in pleasure. Why not? This is it. Don't miss it.

The Eightfold Path doesn't guarantee a perfect life. Nothing does. While I've been on the path, I still continue to experience painful moments, like losing my mom, my two beloved dogs, and watching as one of my daughters returned to a second round of eating disorder treatment after what seemed like a successful year. And I haven't stopped shooting myself with the second arrow entirely.

In my naiveté, I thought that with determination and commitment I would be able to completely transform our multigenerational family patterns of compulsive eating. I think I made a few strides, but I'm okay with passing the baton to my kids. Now that they can make their own decisions, it's their turn to make their own steps in the direction of peace. We have infinite lifetimes to work on this, and nowhere to really get to anyway.

In Japanese culture there is the concept of wabi-sabi, loosely understood as "the beauty of imperfection." It too is based on the same Three Contemplations of dissatisfaction, impermanence, and interbeing. Things can be beautiful in spite of being, or even because they are, imperfect, impermanent, and incomplete. We can celebrate the sincerity, asymmetry, irregularity, simplicity, modesty, and naturalness of our lives and not expect perfection.

My mom, like a lot of us, didn't like to think of herself or any of us as less than perfect, which contributed to some of my childhood feelings of being alone with my suffering. She might not have known how to tolerate distressing emotions and situations, so she avoided them. Like all the rest of us, she just wanted peace. And like me, her strategies didn't always pan out. Just as I've learned to have compassion for my own suffering, I now have compassion for my mom's suffering too.

One of the things my mother did beautifully was look for the good in everything and express enthusiastic, unrestrained excitement, especially for her grandkids. Year after year, Mom showed up at our house in DC with bags full of gifts for our four young kids. She was as excited as they were. The expression on her face as she walked up to the front door was like the face you might see in a photograph of a baby about to blow out the candles on her first birthday cake: eyes and mouth wide open as if to say, "How can so much wonderfulness be mine?!"

Looking for the good in things and unrestrained giving are not my strongest qualities (remember the mango?), so my mom's memory serves as a role model for me. None of us is perfect. It's almost like we need everyone around us in order to make one whole being. My mom was an expert on excitement; I'm pretty good at honesty. And we can each tap into that wholeness when we come into the present moment. When I'm really mindful, my mom and her enthusiasm are here inside me. Grandma's loving hugs are here too, alongside my teacher's wisdom.

The Buddha called this wholeness that's inside each of us "Buddha Nature." It's also known as Self-in-Presence or just Self (with a capital S), and some people I know call it God. I meditate every morning because it keeps me tethered to this wholeness. If I go too long without meditating, I get further away from presence and I start to feel lost; that's when I am most at risk of bingeing or snapping at a loved one. Our Buddha Nature/Self-in-Presence is like a well that sits just beneath the surface of our daily lives. It's full of everything we need to regain our peaceful relationship to food. We can reach it simply by pausing and coming back to our senses. Breathing in, I know I am breathing in. Breathing out, I know I am breathing out.

I had my own wabi-sabi moment while I was writing this book. During the writing of my first draft, I developed a fever for three days, after which

I became so fatigued that I could barely get up off the couch. I canceled all my teaching gigs, including my annual women's mindfulness retreat. Some days I couldn't even walk the dogs.

On the second day of my illness, which lasted for three months, I started to think a lot about meat. I had been ninety-nine percent vegetarian for many years at this point, and had been trying to eat a mostly vegan diet for the previous twenty-four months. But that day I couldn't think of anything but steak. On the third day, my husband went to work, leaving me in my bed exhausted and feverish. The idea of eating meat kept coming into my mind, but it clashed violently with the image I held of myself as a "good" vegetarian Buddhist.

When I turned toward my feelings, I realized that I wasn't being true to my body or my mind. Two years earlier I had read *The Mindful Carnivore: A Vegetarian's Hunt for Sustenance* by Tovar Cerulli and learned that even organic vegetable farms are doing harm, not only to 'pests' like cabbage worms and white-tailed deer but also to species that lived on the land before it was farmed.

There was something in me that wanted to believe that if I could only stay a vegan, I would be free from the guilt of causing harm. But the truth is we can never avoid harming others. We can only do our best to reduce our impact. In my illness I knew I had to consider the harm I was causing myself as well. I picked up the phone and I ordered a big fat Reuben sandwich from the local deli. Because I was sick, I had it delivered to the house, and I ate the whole thing in my bed. I was sad that I had caused harm to the cow, but mostly my body was relieved to have the nutrients it seemed to need at that time. As soon as I ate the sandwich I felt much better.

It's been less than a year since the Reuben, and I am continuing my experiment of eating a small amount of animal food when I feel I need it, which is getting less and less often. In my attempt to reduce the amount of suffering I am causing, this past winter I joined in with a small group of friends to "share a cow." We each got a small portion of a single cow that is raised and slaughtered as humanely as possible. My friend who knows the farmer told me that he cries when he takes the cow's life. I sometimes cry when I eat the meat, but I also give huge thanks to her (I call her Bessie) for helping restore my health. I also know that nothing lasts, so I know this too is another phase. I continue to sit with the paradox that I will never be able to end all animal suffering (whether I choose to eat meat or not) and at the same time I am committed to doing my best not to cause harm. Holding both of these truths is the best I can do right now.

When my daughter Lucile was most actively suffering from her eating disorder, I thought, "If she gets through this, everything will be great." When she left her treatment program, she started back at college with one class. It was slow-going, but over the next three years she caught up to where she needed to be, made new friends, and graduated with honors. It was great. And during those same three years, her sister Veronica had to leave college twice for eating disorder treatment. She too is recovering, slowly.

Still Cooking

The difficulties are not over. They never are, and thank God—because if the difficulties needed to be over before I could stop punishing myself with emotional eating, feeling despair, and getting drunk, I'd be passed out in a food and alcohol coma right now. But I'm not. I'm writing this book so you can know that your relationship with food doesn't have to be perfect for life to be pretty damn good.

No loaf of homemade bread is ever flawless, but most of them are delicious anyway. At first I thought doing meditation and going to Sangha would make me perfect, or at least really "good." It hasn't. I still eat in front of my computer (though not always), and I still eat when I am stressed out (though much less often). I still get angry at my husband, worry about my kids, and feel sad when I lose a good friend.

But here's what is different. Now I can eat a meal without shame. When I do things that aren't healthy for me, rather than beating myself up, I feel compassion for the part of me that wasn't getting her needs met. I'm not angry at food anymore for being so delicious and "making me" eat it. I recognize that I have a choice. When I'm eating a sweet potato and mushroom sandwich, I revel in it. I could be telling myself that I shouldn't eat so much bread, and okay, I sometimes still do. But I know it's a choice.

All four of our kids have matured into the most lovely human beings I could ever want to know, though, like me and so many others, they are still in the process of healing their relationships with food. Paul and I have unique and loving relationships with each one of them. But since I'm no longer blaming myself for all their troubles, I certainly can't take responsibility for their innate and expanding wisdom.

Our children have deep mindfulness roots, though none have strong meditation practices—at least not yet. I see them turn to their mindfulness now and then, especially when they are involved with others who practice or are going through a rocky period. I try not to worry too much about them because I know that my worrying will only prevent me from being here with them in the present moment. And I love being in the present moment with them so much!

When we moved to our current house about eighteen years ago, we decided to host an annual pre-Christmas dinner party just like my family of origin did every December 23. The first year, we invited two families over for a lovely lamb and potato dinner with wine from my husband's collection. The following year we added a few more friends. Year after year, old friends have moved away and new friends have joined, but the core of the group remains.

During the first few years, I cooked a simple dinner at home. In addition to lamb, I usually cooked a vegetarian dish (often it was macaroni and cheese), and when we had lots of really young kids, we ordered pizza for them. As the number of guests grew and we got busier, it started feeling like too much to cook. One year we had it catered by a neighbor, and the next year we made it a potluck. Every family had several kids, who eventually became adults. Our house got crowded, so we moved the party off-site. One year we borrowed a friend's art gallery and had catered food and a DJ. The next year we rented a cycling studio and had a holiday video stream in the background while we ate. The last few years we have served only vegan food.

One year we were too overwhelmed with work and kids to organize the party, and our friends were very disappointed.

This year, the last one in our house because we are moving, we had sixty people for the party. They were Buddhists, Christians, Jews, Muslims, and atheists. Only six were underage. Some we had known since birth, some since college, some only a year or two. Our lives have intertwined in many ways—through work, children, neighborhood, Sangha, and school. We've seen each other go through mental and physical health crises, work changes, marriages, divorces, and the loss of parents. And by some miracle all of us have survived.

I decided to go back to basics and cook the whole damn meal at home. Luckily, I didn't think too much about what might go wrong or how people would judge my food (one of our guests, Rich, was trained at the Ritz Escoffier cooking school in Paris). I just set out to have fun and provide loving nourishment for our friends. We rented a heated tent for the side yard and opened the family room doors to create an enormous dining room.

Going back to basics meant going back to our original meal of baked leg of lamb. Now that I was eating meat periodically, it made sense. The menu also included a grown-up version of macaroni and cheese (heavy on the butter and cream), a vegan main dish (white bean cassoulet), and lots of roasted seasonal root vegetables. We started with two appetizers—Lucile's famous Armenian cheese triangles (which she makes for her own "Friends-giving" dinners now) and Veronica's favorite baked sweet potato fries. We had French onion soup for the first course, and a salad and cheese plate after our mains. Dessert was a variety buffet of sweets brought by guests and some purchased by me at our local farmer's market.

I wanted to choose lamb that had been humanely raised, and I remembered that a neighborhood boy (now a man), who had at different times been the love interest of two daughters (Lucile and Jamie), was now sourcing grass-fed meats from local Maryland and Virginia farms. I called him, and he was able to provide me with five legs of lamb from a Maryland farm that he himself had worked on in the past. (Our friend Mona provided the sixth.) He rode over on his cooler-enhanced bike two days before the party to bring the lamb and give it time to defrost.

I wrote out my plan for the cooking. I had to consider our three gluten-free guests, the five or six vegans, and the several other vegetarians, along with the people who ate it all. I began with the macaroni and cheese—I figured that would keep the longest and heat up well. I lined the pasta boxes up along the counter next to my stove and started boiling water on all the back burners. Only five minutes into my multiday cooking spree I heard an explosion and the sound of glass raining into the kitchen and the family room behind it. The entire glass backsplash behind our stove had exploded, spewing little pieces of glass everywhere. My peacefulness started to slip and my mind spun, "Could I continue to use the stove? Would there be more explosions? Should I give up?"

Without panicking, I cleaned up the glass shards and made sure that nothing got into the open food items. The glass that remained on the wall seemed likely to stay there, so I decided to slowly move forward with my cooking. I just wouldn't use the back burners. The food would take twice as long to prepare, but I could still do it if I stayed focused. I was starting to stress out and in danger of killing the joy of the process, so I reminded myself that my friends would continue to like me even if the food was awful. I didn't have to do this perfectly. If the food was bad, we could always order Indian food.

The rest of that day and the next went pretty well. All four kids were home, and they came into the kitchen to help grate cheese or talk to me about their latest adventures. I enjoyed both the familiar—the kids at home and the smell of the baking cheese—and also the unfamiliar—the flavor of the bean cassoulet and the texture of the gluten-free pasta.

On the day of the party, our chef-trained friend, Rich, dropped by to lend a hand. I was thrilled to have another cook in the kitchen, and he knew just how to make himself useful—he prepared the salad with romaine, arugula, red onions, and thinly sliced watermelon radishes (he was an expert with the mandolin slicer), and he also gave great advice on the lamb. It was nice to feel supported by another cook, and he promised to come into the kitchen to carve the meat when it was time.

Just as the last cassoulet was pulled from the oven, it was time to get dressed for the party. The college students we had hired to help us serve and clean up arrived, they arranged a bar area and helped us set the tables. Our friends began to arrive. Each person took the red paper star with their name written on it to a place setting at one of the six tables. Then they mingled and enjoyed the appetizers and some singing.

When it was time to begin serving the first course—onion soup—I realized that, although I had cooked a batch of gluten-free soup, I had accidently combined it with the rest of the glutinous soup! Our three gluten-free guests got no soup. Next we served the main courses. None of the lamb had been carved yet, so I pulled my husband, Rich, and one of the college kids into the kitchen and pressed upon them to work quickly. Lamb drippings were spilling everywhere while we tried to get the three kinds of macaroni and cheese onto the right tables. We had taken the lamb out a little too early, so some of the pieces were undercooked, but it was too late to fix that, so we served it as it was.

I told one of the servers which dishes were gluten-free macaroni, which were vegan, and which were cheesy regular. They all looked the same. After all the gluten-free and vegan plates had been delivered, I realized that I had made a mistake and had told them the wrong thing. The vegan macaroni had gone to the gluten-free guests and the gluten-free macaroni to the vegan guests. Oh shit! I asked the server to run back out and switch them. She was not amused and grudgingly snatched the plates from the gluten-free guests before they damaged their intestines. The vegans weren't happy either, but soon everyone had their correct plates.

The table of mostly young vegans called out that they didn't have the white bean cassoulet, which for them was the main course. A meat-loving table didn't get their lamb until the rest of their food was finished. We kept our friends entertained with a big glass jar in the center of each table into which each guest added a "gift"—something previously used from their home that had significance—and during dinner each person could pull something interesting out of the jar, have it explained to them, and keep it as their Secret Santa potlatch gift.

By the end of dinner, everyone was full and happy. Salad and cheese plates went off without a hitch. Afterward, we all got up, cleared the tables, and danced. Moms danced with daughters, brothers with sisters, and young with old. The old folks had all said good-bye by midnight, but the young ones stayed up for a few more hours.

The meal was far from perfect. It was big and messy and we made a lot of mistakes. I did my best to satisfy everyone's individual needs, though I accepted in advance that not everyone would be happy. I felt great. I had been able to give a gift to our cherished friends, who had given us so much over the years. My mother was there in spirit, because I was inspired to give without expecting much in return. I certainly wasn't breathing mindfully the whole time I was cooking or serving or eating. But I was aware that it was a very precious moment, one that will never happen again. And I took a chance. I let myself risk showing my messy, imperfect cooking and my messy, imperfect self.

Chogyam Trungpa Rinpoche said, "Real fearlessness is the product of tenderness. It comes from letting the world tickle your heart, your raw and beautiful heart. You are willing to open up, without resistance or shyness, and face the world. You are willing to share your heart with others."

One thing I have learned since beginning this journey is that all of us just want happiness and peace. Those of us who get caught in addictions of any kind really wish we could be free of it—we just don't know how. Mindfulness offered me a path to freedom. I can live with myself as I am— fat, skinny, messy, pimply, loved, unloved, too busy, too lazy, good cook, or crappy cook—because none of those judgments are real.

Mindfulness takes us beyond all the dualistic notions of fat or skinny, good cook or bad cook, good parent or bad parent. We're just here and this is it. When we arrive in this very moment, breathing it in through our senses, none of these judgments even make sense. We can embrace the moment and share it with others. Nothing else really matters.

Baked Sweet Potato Fries *(vegan)*

This is one of Veronica's favorite foods—she likes them made with simply olive oil and salt.

INGREDIENTS:

- 3 sweet potatoes, cut into strips
- 2 to 3 tablespoons olive or other oil
- ½ teaspoon smoked paprika, cumin, Old Bay Seasoning, pepper, or other seasonsings as you like
- 1 teaspoon salt

METHOD:

Preheat oven to 425 degrees.

Wash and cut sweet potatoes into strips.

Place sweet potato strips in a bowl with the olive oil, salt, and any other spices you choose. Mix well.

Spread the sweet potato strips on a baking sheet so they're not touching.

Bake in the top half of the oven for 20 minutes, or until brown and soft.

Serves 4 to 6.

Grandma's Homemade Bread (vegan option)

This recipe is based on the original given to me while I watched my Grandma baking it only a few months before she passed away in 1989. My memory of watching her bake is very precious. Her kitchen was simple, and she rolled and kneaded her bread right on her old kitchen table. She worked consciously and always had a sweet smile on her face. She was slightly embarrassed by all my questions. To her, making bread was something anyone could do. I hope you find that sense of ease carried forward from my grandma as you bake it for yourself and your family. For more details on making the bread, reread the first section of chapter 8.

Honey isn't technically vegan, so I have offered a substitute. Do what makes you feel comfortable.

INGREDIENTS:

5 cups hot water

1 heaping tablespoon salt

8 to 10 cups unbleached white flour

1 stick (¼ pound) margarine (Grandma used Fleischmann's. I use Earth Balance soy margarine or real butter.)

½ cup honey or agave syrup

2 packages quick-rising yeast

⅛ cup dry milk (for vegan version, use nutritional yeast or leave out)

METHOD:

Combine the water, salt, and margarine, and let stand until the margarine is melted and the water is room temperature.

Add the yeast to the water mixture. Let stand a few more minutes until bubbly. (Note: If it doesn't get bubbly, the yeast may be too old. Try again with new yeast.)

Sift together nutritional yeast with a small amount of flour and mix into the liquids.

Continue adding flour until the dough becomes thick. Then beat it by hand or with a Kitchen Aid or other heavy-duty mixer.

Keep adding flour until you can't add any more.

Roll out the dough on a floured surface, like a countertop.

Knead the dough and continue adding flour until it becomes smooth and elastic, about 10 minutes. Form the dough into a ball.

Grease a large bowl and place the ball of dough into the bowl. Flip the dough over so both sides are greased.

Cover the bowl with a towel, and leave in a warm place for the dough to rise, until it's about double its original size. This may take 2 to 4 hours.

Punch the dough down everywhere on its surface. Flip it over and let it rise again, another 2 to 4 hours.

Take the dough out of the bowl and cut it into 5 pieces.

Roll out each piece like a snake; tuck the ends under, and place into a greased bread pan.

Cover and let it rise one more time.

Bake on the middle rack of a preheated 350 degree oven for about 30 minutes.

The bread is done when it has browned and when knocking it on the bottom makes a hollow sound.

Makes 5 to 6 loaves.

Appendices

The Five Mindfulness Trainings

The First Mindfulness Training: Reverence for Life

Aware of the suffering caused by the destruction of life, I am committed to cultivating the insight of interbeing and compassion and learning ways to protect the lives of people, animals, plants, and minerals. I am determined not to kill, not to let others kill, and not to support any act of killing in the world, in my thinking, or in my way of life. Seeing that harmful actions arise from anger, fear, greed, and intolerance, which in turn come from dualistic and discriminative thinking, I will cultivate openness, nondiscrimination, and nonattachment to views in order to transform violence, fanaticism, and dogmatism in myself and in the world.

The Second Mindfulness Training: True Happiness

Aware of the suffering caused by exploitation, social injustice, stealing, and oppression, I am committed to practicing generosity in my thinking, speaking, and acting. I am determined not to steal and not to possess anything that should belong to others; and I will share my time, energy, and material resources with those who are in need. I will practice looking deeply to see that the happiness and suffering of others are not separate from my own happiness and suffering; that true happiness is not possible without understanding and compassion; and that running after wealth, fame, power, and sensual pleasures can bring much suffering and despair. I am aware that happiness depends on my mental attitude and not on external conditions, and that I can live happily in the present moment simply by remembering that I already have more than enough conditions to be happy. I am committed to practicing Right Livelihood so that I can help reduce the suffering of living beings on Earth and reverse the process of global warming.

The Third Mindfulness Training: True Love

Aware of the suffering caused by sexual misconduct, I am committed to cultivating responsibility and learning ways to protect the safety and integrity of individuals, couples, families, and society. Knowing that sexual desire is not love, and that sexual activity motivated by craving always harms myself as well as others, I am determined not to engage in sexual relations without true love and a deep, long-term commitment made known to my family and friends. I will do everything in my power to protect children from sexual abuse and to prevent couples and families from being broken by sexual misconduct. Seeing that body and mind are one, I am committed to learning appropriate ways to take care of my sexual energy and cultivating loving kindness, compassion, joy and inclusiveness—which are the four basic elements of true love—for my greater happiness and the greater happiness of others. Practicing true love, we know that we will continue beautifully into the future.

The Fourth Mindfulness Training: Loving Speech and Deep Listening

Aware of the suffering caused by unmindful speech and the inability to listen to others, I am committed to cultivating loving speech and compassionate listening in order to relieve suffering and to promote reconciliation and peace in myself and among other people, ethnic and religious groups, and nations. Knowing that words can create happiness or suffering, I am committed to speaking truthfully using words that inspire confidence, joy, and hope. When anger is manifesting in me, I am determined not to speak.

I will practice mindful breathing and walking in order to recognize and to look deeply into my anger. I know that the roots of anger can be found in my wrong perceptions and lack of understanding of the suffering in myself and in the other person. I will speak and listen in a way that can help myself and the other person to transform suffering and see the way out of difficult situations. I am determined not to spread news that I do not know to be certain and not to utter words that can cause division or discord. I will practice Right Diligence to nourish my capacity for understanding, love, joy, and inclusiveness, and gradually transform anger, violence, and fear that lie deep in my consciousness.

The Fifth Mindfulness Training: Nourishment and Healing

Aware of the suffering caused by unmindful consumption, I am committed to cultivating good health, both physical and mental, for myself, my family, and my society by practicing mindful eating, drinking, and consuming. I will practice looking deeply into how I consume the Four Kinds of Nutriments, namely edible foods, sense impressions, volition, and consciousness. I am determined not to gamble, or to use alcohol, drugs, or any other products that contain toxins, such as certain websites, electronic games, TV programs, films, magazines, books, and conversations. I will practice coming back to the present moment to be in touch with the refreshing, healing, and nourishing elements in me and around me, not letting regrets and sorrow drag me back into the past nor letting anxieties, fear, or craving pull me out of the present moment. I am determined not to try to cover up loneliness, anxiety, or other suffering by losing myself in consumption. I will contemplate interbeing and consume in a way that preserves peace, joy, and well-being in my body and consciousness, and in the collective body and consciousness of my family, my society, and the Earth.

The Five Contemplations

To recite before eating:

This food is a gift of the earth, the sky, numerous living beings, and much hard and loving work.

May we eat with mindfulness and gratitude so as to be worthy to receive this food.

May we recognize and transform unwholesome mental formations, especially our greed and learn to eat with moderation.

May we keep our compassion alive by eating in such a way that reduces the suffering of living beings, stops contributing to climate change, and heals and preserves our precious planet.

We accept this food so that we may nurture our brotherhood and sisterhood, build our Sangha, and nourish our ideal of serving all living beings.

Froglessness

The first fruition of the practice
is the attainment of froglessness.

When a frog is put
on the center of a plate,
she will jump out of the plate
after just a few seconds.

If you put the frog back again
on the center of the plate,
she will again jump out.

You have so many plans.
There is something you want to become.
Therefore you always want to make a leap,
a leap forward.

It is difficult
to keep the frog still
on the center of the plate.
You and I
both have Buddha Nature in us.
This is encouraging,
but you and I
both have Frog Nature in us.

That is why
the first attainment
of the practice—
froglessness is its name.

How to Find Your Own Mindfulness Community

As I explain in chapter 7, finding a mindfulness community was one of the most important pieces of my healing from bulimia and compulsive eating. There are communities in the Plum Village Zen tradition in which I practice, but don't feel that you need to limit yourself to these. There are groups practicing all over the world in all kinds of traditions. They meet in yoga studios, temples, church halls, and people's living rooms.

If you can't find a community that feels comfortable, it's easy to start your own. Just ask a friend or two to come over and do sitting meditation with you every week, every two weeks, or even every month (though it's harder to keep momentum when you meet less than every two weeks). You can follow the plan below to structure your time, or simply use the time to share about the joys and challenges of your mindfulness practices, whether formal practices—like sitting and walking meditation—or informal practices, like mindful cooking, eating, speaking, and listening.

Links for Finding a Sangha in Your Area:

Meditation in the Plum Village tradition:
  http://iamhome.org/directory/
Christian meditation:
  http://wccm-usa.org/about-meditation/finding-a-meditation-group/
Local meditation groups may be listed as Meetup groups:
  www.meetup.com

Getting Started with Your Own Weekly or Biweekly Sangha:

1. Gather in a circle. You can sit on cushions, blankets, or furniture.

2. Choose someone to be in charge of timing. If you have a small bell, the timer can invite the bell three times to indicate the beginning of the meditation.

3. We usually sit together for twenty minutes at a time (but you could decide to do less if you are short on time).

4. After twenty minutes, the timer invites the bell two times to indicate that the sitting meditation is over.

5. If you'd like, you can do walking meditation for ten to fifteen minutes. Walking meditation is just like sitting, in that you keep bringing your mind back to the present moment except instead of paying attention to your breath, you pay attention to your steps (see Thich Nhat Hanh's book *Happiness* for a description of walking meditation).

6. After completing your meditation time, you can read a short piece from a mindfulness-related book that you like (Thich Nhat Hanh, Sylvia Boorstein, and Sharon Salzberg's books provide short readings that we have found useful). Each person can read a paragraph or two, and afterward you can have a short discussion about your practice and how the reading relates to what you are going through right now.

7. The time keeper can let the group know when you are getting near the end of your prearranged end time, and can invite the bell to close the session.

Notes

1. Jennifer L. Harris, John A. Bargh, and Kelly D. Brownell, "Priming Effects of Television Food Advertising on Eating Behavior," *Health Psychology,* 2009 Jul; 28(4): 404–413, accessed April 19, 2015, http://www.ncbi.nlm.nih.gov/pmc/articles/PMC2743554/.

2. Alan Watts, *The Wisdom of Insecurity: A Message for an Age of Anxiety* (New York: Vintage Books, 2011), 116.

3. "Embodied Situated Cognition/The Felt Sense," *Embodiment Resources,* accessed April 19, 2015, http://www.embodiment.org.uk/topics/felt_sense.htm.

4. William Stierle, "Marshall Rosenberg's Nonviolent Communication (NVC)," *Yogi Times,* accessed April 19, 2015, http://www.yogitimes.com/article/marshall-rosenberg-NVC-non-violent-communication.

5. Norman Fischer, "Suzuki Roshi's Way," *DharmaNet International,* accessed April 19, 2015, http://www.dharmanet.org/suzukirway.htm.

6. Kathleen D. Vohs, Yajin Wang, Francesca Gino, and Michael I. Norton, "Rituals Enhance Consumption," *Psychological Science,* July 17, 2013, accessed May 7, 2015, http://pss.sagepub.com/content/early/2013/07/17/0956797613478949.abstract.

7. Anne-Marie Mouly and Regina Sullivan, "Chapter 15: Memory and Plasticity in the Olfactory System: From Infancy to Adulthood," *The Neurobiology of Olfaction* (Boca Raton, FL: CRC Press, 2010), http://www.ncbi.nlm.nih.gov/books/NBK55967/#ch15_r91.

8. Bijal P. Trivedi, "Neuroscience: Hardwired for Taste," *Nature* 486, no. 7403 (2012): S7–S9, http://www.nature.com/nature/journal/v486/n7403_supp/full/486S7a.html.

9. Burkhard Bilger, "The Possibilian," *New Yorker,* April 25, 2011, http://www.newyorker.com/magazine/2011/04/25/the-possibilian.

10. Bhikkhu Bodhi, *In the Buddha's Words: An Anthology of Discourses from the Pali Canon* (Somerville, MA: Wisdom Publications, 2005), 63–64.

11. Bhikkhu Bodhi, "Setting in Motion the Wheel of the Dhamma," *BuddhaSasana*, accessed April 19, 2015, http://www.budsas.org/ebud/ebsut001.htm.

12. "Americans Eat Out about Five Times a Week," *United Press International*, September 19, 2011, http://www.upi.com/Health_News/2011/09/19/Americans-eat-out-about-5-times-a-week/54241316490172/.

13. Lindsey P. Smith, Shu Wen Ng, and Barry M. Popkin, "Trends in US Home Food Preparation and Consumption: Analysis of National Nutrition Surveys and Time Use Studies from 1965–1966 to 2007–2008," *Nutrition Journal* 12 (2013): 45, http://www.ncbi.nlm.nih.gov/pmc/articles/PMC3639863/.

14. "Residential Energy Consumption Survey (RECS)," *U.S. Energy Information Association*, accessed April 19, 2015, http://www.eia.gov/consumption/residential/data/2009/.

15. Scott Darnell, "Forced to Sit," *Lion's Roar: Buddhist Wisdom for Our Time*, November 1, 2008, http://www.lionsroar.com/forced-to-sit/.

16. Reed Larson and Craig Johnson, "Bulimia: Disturbed Patterns of Solitude," *Addictive Behaviors* 10, no. 3 (1985): 281–290, http://www.sciencedirect.com/science/article/pii/0306460385900097.

17. Bruce K. Alexander, "Addiction: The View from Rat Park," brucekalexander.com, accessed April 19, 2015, http://www.brucekalexander.com/articles-speeches/177-addiction-the-view-from-rat-park-2.

18. "Kalyāṇa-mittatā," *Wikipedia*, last modified January 20, 2015, http://en.wikipedia.org/wiki/Kaly%C4%81%E1%B9%87a-mittat%C4%81.

19. Chris Jones, "Vince Vaughn: The Biggest Man in the Room," *Esquire*, November 18, 2008, accessed May 7, 2015, http://www.esquire.com/news-politics/a5285/vince-vaughn-1208/.

20. Rex Reed, "Declined: In Identity Thief, Bateman's Bankable Billing Can't Lift This Flick Out of the Red," *Observer*, February 5, 2013, accessed May 7, 2015, http://observer.com/2013/02/declined-in-identity-thief-batemans-bankable-billing-cant-lift-this-flick-out-of-the-red/.

21. Phillip Moffitt, "How Suffering Got a Bad Name," *Huffington Post*, last modified November 17, 2011, http://www.huffingtonpost.com/phillip-moffitt/how-suffering-got-a-bad-n_b_105620.html.

Acknowledgments

Because of the truth of interdependence, all beneficial aspects of this book arise from our collective knowing. Any unwholesome aspects most likely came from what remains unskillful or unhealed in me.

There were so many people who made this book possible, starting with my parents and all of my ancestors. My mom's dedication to combining faith and social justice is the heartbeat of my life, and my dad's creative and emotional expression and uncompromising freedom give me the space I need to learn and grow. My grandma Lucile's nurturing lives on in me whenever I step into the kitchen or serve a meal. I am grateful to have been cooked in the same pot with my brother and sisters who inspire me in the many fierce ways they serve and heal.

The idea for writing this book came from my dear friend Sister Pine without whom I would not have had this opportunity. Of course, without my teacher, Thich Nhat Hanh, from whom I learned most of what I understand about life, I would never have known Sister Pine. Had I not attended the Angeles Arrien retreat, I might not have known about Thich Nhat Hanh. And without my friend Deidre, I wouldn't have known about Angeles' retreat. You see how this list includes everyone, including you, the reader. I am because we are.

I interviewed and chatted with dozens of people about this book and I thank you all. Even if you don't show up in the pages, you influenced what and how I wrote. Because of space limitations, not every recipe contributed could fit here, but I have tried them all and am grateful for your generosity. Special thanks to my first editors and cheerleaders, Martha Bullen and Paul Mahon who never doubted I could do this, even when I whined about it. To my editors at Parallax—Debra Ollivier, the mysterious JEK, and especially Rachel Neumann—thank you for teaching me how to write a book. The rest of the team at Parallax has been invaluable as well, including Nancy Fish, Jason Kim, and Terry Barber.

In addition to Thich Nhat Hanh, I am grateful for the profound wisdom revealed to me by Roshi Joan Halifax, whose fire lights the way toward serving all beings; Phillip Moffitt, who holds all of us students of the dharma in his deep intention toward liberation; Marshall Rosenberg, who taught me how to curse with compassion; Mitchell Ratner, my favorite dharma sparring partner and a humble but incredibly dedicated mindfulness teacher who is always smiling like a Buddha; Anh-Huong and Thu Nguyen who present an example of truly mindful living; and Sharon Salzberg, Pema Chodron, Linji, Dogen, and all of my other dharma ancestors.

I have had many amazing yoga teachers and body workers over the years who were instrumental in helping me reconcile with my body, including Kate Miller, Robin Carnes, Suzie Hurley, Gail Harris, Luann Fortune, Sarah Lawrie, and the ones whose names I don't remember now. Thanks to all of the teachers at Howard University School of Divinity, especially Cheryl J. Sanders, Dr. Cain Hope Felder, and Dr. Kelly Brown Douglas, for challenging me on my ethics, spirituality, and race biases.

My understanding of my own mind was also supported by spending time in therapy with two of the most professional, compassionate, and uncompromising therapists: Dr. Samuel Lashley and Dr. Linda Moore. They helped me untie many knots. Ann Weiser Cornell has been a guide through these waters as well by teaching me how to untie the knots myself using Inner Relationship Focusing.

My first BFF, Sharon Rakowski deserves acknowledgment for taking me under her wing when I was a twelve-year-old bookish burnout. As a Facebook friend (even though we lost touch nearly forty years ago) she replied enthusiastically to my post about this book, "That's so great, you always wanted to write a book!" And my friend Yo Chin who helped guide me back toward healthy eating and living when I was lost. Special gratitude to my many sister-friends who inspire and encourage me, including Deidre Combs, Julie Causey, Camille Martone, Julia Jarvis and Karen Coley.

Thanks to Colman McCarthy and Marsha Blakeway for being the first people to show me how to share what I was learning with my community.

My friends in the Thich Nhat Hanh meditation Sangha are the cornerstone of my mindfulness. I learn something from every single person I meet on a retreat or meditation event. I bow to Lynda and David Martin-McCormick, Lynd Morris, Sister Pine, Mary Carnell, Marie Sheppard, Mick Neustadt, Maria Sgamboti, Kaira Jewel, Susan Hadler, Jindra Cekan, Barbra Esher, Wonder, Ben King, Suki Fredericks, and every member of the Opening Heart Mindfulness and Still Water mindfulness communities.

Every single adult or child who came through the doors of Circle Yoga and my mindfulness classes and those who read my blog taught me how to communicate about mindfulness. And I owe a huge debt of gratitude to the women who believed in my vision for sharing mindfulness with the DC community, especially Linda Feldman, Gayle Hager, Anne Kennedy, Penny Bell, Sarah Brown, and Debra Person-Mishalove.

My four children are the reason I care. I don't think they could possibly bring me any more joy (and tears) than they do. I adore them and am especially grateful for their honesty, love, and bravery and their willingness to let me tell their stories along with mine. I can clearly see how the practice of mindfulness shows up in each of their lives.

My sister, Julie, and my husband, Paul, are my rocks. They have managed to love me long enough to slice through the certainty of my unlovableness. I know my life is altogether different than it would have been without them, yet all I can offer them is my unending gratitude.

Related Titles from Parallax Press

Awakening Joy, James Baraz and Shoshana Alexander

Carrot in the Cosmos, Carmen Yuen

Healing, Sister Dang Nghiem

How to Eat, Thich Nhat Hanh

No Mud No Lotus, Thich Nhat Hanh

Not Quite Nirvana, Rachel Neumann

Reconciliation, Thich Nhat Hanh

Small Bites, Annabelle Zinser

Ten Breaths to Happiness, Glen Schneider

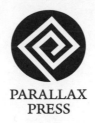

PARALLAX
PRESS

Parallax Press is a nonprofit publisher, founded and inspired by Zen Master Thich Nhat Hanh. We publish books on mindfulness in daily life and are committed to making these teachings accessible to everyone and preserving them for future generations. We do this work to alleviate suffering and contribute to a more just and joyful world.

For a copy of the catalog, please contact:

Parallax Press
P.O. Box 7355
Berkeley, CA 94707
(510) 540-6411
parallax.org

The author's royalties from sales of the book will be contributed to organizations sharing the practices of mindful cooking and eating.